THE YEAR OF *Sarah*

Oprah,

    Thank you for your inspiration and for lifting other's voices!

You inspire me to do the same ♡

xo Sarah

FROM HEARTBROKEN TO HAPPY
AND THE LONG DISTANCE IN BETWEEN

THE YEAR OF
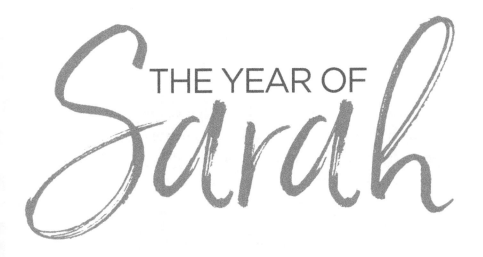

SARAH DEBLOCK

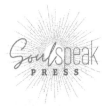

©2025 by Sarah DeBlock
All rights reserved.

No part of this publication may be reproduced or transmitted in any form or by any means, electronic or mechanical, including photography, recording, or any information storage and retrieval system, without permission in writing from the author.

Requests for permission to make copies of any part of the work should be emailed to the following email address: info@jessbuchanan.com.

Published and distributed by Soul Speak Press
Virginia, USA

Cover photograph by Renée C. Gage

Library of Congress Control Number: 2024926321
DeBlock, Sarah

The Year of Sarah: From Heartbroken to Happy and the Long Distance In Between

ISBN 978-1-958472-13-2 Paperback
ISBN 978-1-958472-14-9 eBook

To all brave souls who have ever loved deeply

To all fearless individuals searching to heal

To my partner and life-long teacher Ryan

To my yoga guru Padma Shakti, who encouraged me to share my story.

Contents

Foreword . . . 1

Letter to the Reader . . . 5

PART ONE · BREAKING . . . 9

ONE
The Dreaded Day . . . 11

TWO
How It Started . . . 13

THREE
First Day . . . 27

FOUR
Sundays . . . 31

FIVE
A Year . . . 37

SIX
Type A . . . 39

SEVEN
Criticism . . . 45

EIGHT
Phone Calls . . . 53

NINE
Failure . . . 59

TEN
Then . . . 63

ELEVEN
Year of Me 67

PART TWO · PAIN 75

TWELVE
Heartburn 79

THIRTEEN
Not Equal 85

FOURTEEN
Falling Foolishly 89

FIFTEEN
Learning to Fail 93

SIXTEEN
Wedding Day 97

SEVENTEEN
Loneliness 107

EIGHTEEN
Second Heartbreak 113

NINETEEN
Truth 119

PART THREE · HEALING 125

TWENTY
Finding Yoga 127

TWENTY-ONE
Rasa Yoga 135

TWENTY-TWO
Change in Consciousness 143

TWENTY-THREE
Sing and Dance 151

TWENTY-FOUR Konnichiwa	155
TWENTY-FIVE Heard	159
TWENTY-SIX Hurricane Harvey	163
TWENTY-SEVEN Papa	175
TWENTY-EIGHT Hiroshima	181
TWENTY-NINE Guilty	187
THIRTY Follow	191
THIRTY-ONE Life is Short	195
PART FOUR · HEALED	**201**
THIRTY-TWO Four Days	203
THIRTY-THREE Flow	209
THIRTY-FOUR Dockweiler	217
THIRTY-FIVE On Call	221
THIRTY-SIX Reunited and Alone	227
THIRTY-SEVEN Dreams	235

THIRTY-EIGHT
Bliss   239

THIRTY-NINE
Virginia   243

FORTY
What if?   249

FORTY-ONE
Friends   251

FORTY-TWO
Breaking Free   253

FORTY-THREE
Third Heartbreak   257

FORTY-FOUR
Settled   263

PART FIVE · CLOSING REFLECTIONS   269

FORTY-FIVE
Opposites Heal   271

Afterword   277

Acknowledgments   279

> Real character is the willingness to make personal sacrifices for a higher ideal. It's the willingness to embrace those ideals that we hold sacred even in the face of temptation and fear.
>
> —RADHANATH SWAMI

Foreword

In an age where isolation can feel suffocating, the act of storytelling becomes a lifeline. It creates space for connection, understanding, and empathy, reminding us that we are never truly alone. One of the most profound truths that emerges from *The Year of Sarah* is the importance of sharing our narratives.

As you read her words, I encourage you to reflect on your own experiences—the moments that have shaped you, the love that has lifted you, and the losses that have taught you the most. It is through this introspection that we forge deeper connections with ourselves and others. *The Year of Sarah* is a heartfelt memoir that chronicles a transformative journey through love, loss, and self-discovery. Written by my devoted student Sarah, this book is not just a story—it is a testament to the resilience of the human spirit and the incredible power of vulnerability in the healing process.

From the moment we met, I admired Sarah's rare and unwavering devotion to true studentship. Her extraordinary spirit, compassionate heart, and profound ability to reflect on her experiences set her apart as a remarkable student and an extraordinary human being. Her constant pursuit of deepening her understanding of Rasa Yoga—embracing it not merely as a physical discipline but as a holistic way of life—has been inspiring to witness. Her commitment to self-growth and healing is not just a personal endeavor; it is a shining light that illuminates every aspect of her life, beautifully captured in this narrative.

Sarah embodies the essence of a born student, embracing the vicissitudes of life with grace and resilience as part of her commitment to consistent growth. In a world rife with codependency, she has steadfastly pursued the healthiest of relationships, choosing connection over attachment and understanding over expectation. It has been an immense privilege to walk this journey with her over these past years. I have been humbled to share my reflections here, conscious of the profound story that lies within these pages—a story few have had the privilege to witness, and one I am honored to convey.

In *The Year of Sarah*, we are apprised of a pivotal year in her life—a time marked by profound heartbreak in a long-distance relationship. It is crucial to understand that this heartbreak, while perhaps different in severity from other challenges one might face, is nonetheless a significant and deeply emotional experience. It reshaped her understanding of love, identity, and human connection. Through her elegant prose, Sarah invites us into the myriad emotions that accompany separation, illustrating that love's complexities can evoke feelings of joy, sorrow, and everything in between.

In the pages that follow, you will embark on a journey that resonates with anyone who has ever loved deeply. As Sarah bravely recounts the evolution of her relationship with Ryan, we witness the beautiful highs and daunting lows that define their time apart. With each word, she paints a vivid picture of the challenges faced—a struggle that demands both introspection and courage. Sarah shows us that even in separation, love remains a powerful force that can illuminate the darkest corners of our hearts.

This memoir is not simply a chronicle of grief; it is an exploration of resilience. It reflects the universal plight of wanting to find ourselves while navigating the often tumultuous waters of relationships. As Sarah delves into her experiences, she reveals how yoga became a sanctuary—a tool for grounding herself during times of uncertainty and emotional upheaval. Through mindfulness and self-reflection, she learns that the journey to happiness is often paved with challenges that force us to confront our true selves.

The Year of Sarah is dedicated to all brave souls who have dared to love and those who are fearless in their search for healing. Sarah's reflections serve as an anchor, offering insights that can help you navigate your own journey. She beautifully articulates the essence of human experience, revealing that we are all intricately connected by our shared struggles and triumphs.

Sarah's story fills our hearts with hope. While she navigates the pain of separation, she also reveals the beauty of rediscovering joy amid heartbreak. It is a poignant reminder that within every challenge lies the seed of growth, waiting for the right conditions to bloom. Her realization that staying joyful in the face of adversity is not only possible but essential is a powerful message for us all.

As you journey through Sarah's experiences, I hope you find inspiration in her strength and vulnerability. May her reflections encourage you to embrace your own trials, celebrate your growth, and continually reaffirm your belief in love's transformative power. Remember that healing does not follow a linear path, and sometimes the most profound shifts occur in the quiet moments of aloneness.

I invite you to immerse yourself in *The Year of Sarah*. Allow her story to resonate within you, guiding you toward your own transformative moments. Let it inspire you to embrace the intricacies of your heart, confront your fears, and embark on a journey toward joy. May you emerge from these pages with a renewed sense of hope, understanding, and a deeper connection to your own truth.

With all my love and blessings,

Padma Shakti

Founder, Rasa Yoga School of Ayurveda Yoga

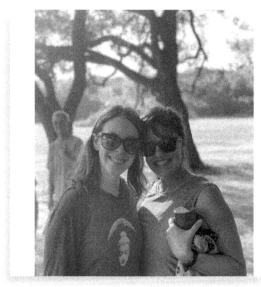

Padma and Sarah at the end of a yoga retreat in Austin, Texas.

Letter to the Reader

To the readers willing to share in my story:

I wrote this book with the hope that at least one person who may be going through a similar situation can learn from my story and suffer less than I did. This reason perplexed some friends and publishers when I told them what I was going to write about, but at the end of the day, this is my Truth. Most books are written to establish credibility or to make money, but honestly, this book's purpose is neither of those. I never fathomed writing a book, despite my long list of dreams, until my yoga teacher encouraged me to share my story for everyone else going through a similar situation. I do believe hearing others' stories is healing, which is why I love reading memoirs. I know many of us share common wounds, and if any of my past resonates with you, I believe reading this book will be worthwhile.

This is a story of a long-distance relationship that led me through the four stages of grief. I struggled immensely after having to live in a different state than my other half. I felt deep heartbreak despite there not being any break up. You may pick up this book and wonder, "What is the big deal about a long-distance relationship? There are so many worse hardships in the world." Yes, you are right, it is not even a trauma, and I would not have guessed I would have taken this news so hard myself. But love and intimate relationships are a funny thing that are at the core of human growth. They can really capture us, and when separated we can feel pain as if half our identity has been stripped from us. There's a reason we love to hear a good love story and that love stories are tales as old as time. This story is one of heartbreak from a long-distance relationship, but that is really just the context and the story is more layered. There were a series of events that made the situation more painful for me; to understand them, it would help for you to know a little bit more about me.

When I was in high school, people would have described me as kind, shy, soft-spoken, and always smiling. My classmates would have told you that I was not in the popular group but that I had a small group of close friends and that my boyfriend and I seemed pretty serious. The popular kids may not have even known me, but I knew everyone because I was always observing everything around me, and I was especially attuned to everyone's emotions. This helped me be a straight A student because I knew exactly what each teacher wanted, and I made sure to meet their expectations. It also hindered me and often led me to be indecisive, since I was summing up how my decision would impact everyone else's mood before considering what I wanted.

As a child, I learned how to note everyone's emotions, and I felt deep sadness with what I witnessed. Most adults I knew were unhappy, including my teachers who complained about their jobs. I also made note that this perpetual discontent revolved around people's jobs, resulting in living for the weekend. This concerned me as I approached the time to start choosing a college major and feared that I, too, would be unhappy as an adult. I wanted to stay joyful. I had no idea how to do this, but as I filled out college essays, I made a strong promise to myself that I would figure that out and be a happy adult.

I had the hardest time choosing what to major in at college. I really did not know what I wanted and this decision weighed heavily on me. Growing up, I had always been involved in a lot of activities. After school, I was part of a dance group, competed in tennis, had started a Go Green club to promote sustainability, and took lessons in piano, painting, voice, and viola. In my senior year, I had even started modeling and being an extra in the background of movies. I loved being part of a variety of things and choosing a major felt like I was pinning myself down to one thing and giving up all the other aspects of life. It was terrifying as a seventeen-year-old and choosing one major felt suffocating.

I did not make my decision quickly, to say the least. It was essentially a process of elimination. The only thing I really knew was that I had a passion for sustainability, and my strengths lied in chemistry and math. This all fit in well with chemical engineering, and as my mom majored in this too, she suggested that I try it. Both of my parents are engineers, and so I surrendered to the fact that it may be in my genes. My parents assured me it would give me many opportunities out of college. I hung onto this and kept reminding myself that I was not putting myself in a box. There was time to find my way.

After I graduated from college, I had not gained much clarity on how I wanted to spend my life. But I had not forgotten my promise to myself that I would figure out how to be a happy adult. I had started practicing yoga in college, which I felt an instant attraction to. It seemed connected to my promise of following a path toward joy, and I knew I wanted to learn more. The high school boyfriend that people would have told you seemed serious, was still my best friend. He always made me smile, and I envisioned him by my side as we figured out life. This was one way in which the separation with long distance was so crushing—it felt like my life was going in the opposite direction of discovering fulfillment. Now I was going out into the corporate working world by myself with the fear of never wanting to respond "I'm living the dream!" sarcastically when asked, "How is it going?"

This is a more universal story, of a young girl right out of college, trying to find herself, holding her convictions to a dream that it was possible to know what it is to be happy. I am now grateful for the winding journey I did not desire, because it brought up some of my deepest fears. They tore me down and forced me to rebuild myself. Through it all, I practiced yoga, which helped me learn that staying joyful in the midst of painful heartbreak is possible. While there are many stories interwoven throughout the chapters of this book, the fundamental truth is that this is really a story of heartbreak and healing; heartbreak caused by the separation I experienced from myself, and the healing path I took to find my voice, let go of pleasing people, and listen to my own heart.

xo Sarah

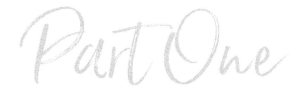

Breaking

*Love knows not its own depths
until its hour of separation.*

—KHALIL GIBRAN, *THE PROPHET*

The lunch bell rang and so began the mad dash when everyone hurried up the stairs from the cafeteria back to class. As I began my trek to seventh grade math class, my body suddenly jolted forward as someone stepped on the back of my left flip-flop. Faster than I could process what was happening, I fell forward and my hands planted perfectly on the butt of the boy in front of me to catch my fall. There was no way he was going to believe this was an accident with how symmetrically they landed on each cheek. My own cheeks instantly turned beet red. I was mortified. The boy turned around with the most confused face—probably checking to see if this was some sort of prank. I looked up. It was Ryan. The only thing I knew about him was his name. I quickly said sorry and looked behind me to retrieve my flip-flop among the stampede of middle schoolers flying up the stairs. My face climbed in temperature as I finished this walk of shame to the top of the stairwell.

Ryan made a right, so I quickly took a left and never looked back. Many years later, I would learn that Ryan has no recollection of this event that was so traumatic for seventh-grade Sarah.

One

The Dreaded Day

I gave Ryan one last hug. "I love you. Have a great first day of grad school. Go show them how amazing you are." I wanted our parting words to be that of encouragement.

"Thanks, babe. I love you too," he replied. After a lingering pause he kept talking, "Okay, I have to go. I'll see you before you know it." He made this statement with a confidence that we both knew was only an attempt to reassure us both.

I closed the door as he waved goodbye and left for his first day of classes at UCLA. Turning to face the inside of his new dorm room with my back to the door, I gazed at all of his familiar belongings—a forest green comforter making up his bed, a small Dirt Devil vacuum cleaner attached to the charger near the closet door, a Doctor Who coffee mug in the corner of his desk, used as a pencil holder—now placed neatly in this unfamiliar setting. I scanned the room and my eyes landed on my already packed pink luggage beside the small couch. I checked my phone for the time; I still had three hours before I needed to leave for my flight and my mind was spinning; it was too painful thinking about the fact that he wouldn't be back before I had to leave. I had never felt so untethered in my life. I couldn't focus on anything. I was facing not only the day, but the exact moment I had been dreading, and denying, if I was being honest, for the last six months. I couldn't stay in this room for three hours without him. Heart pounding, I grabbed my things and hurried to the airport shuttle as quickly as I could. As I watched Los Angeles pass me by from my window of the shuttle, the blur of trees, buildings, and people all seemed to perfectly match how I was experiencing the world at that moment.

As I arrived at the airport, the white lights, tiles, and floors seemed particularly bright and were anything but comforting. I scanned the wall of screens and caught a hard breath of relief when I read there was an earlier flight to Houston. This was happening whether I liked it or not, so catching an earlier flight would reduce the dreadful waiting. I asked the attendant to switch flights and in less than an hour from leaving his room, I found myself in a middle seat in the last row of a Boeing 787 headed east to my new home. A seat I would normally avoid at all costs beat waiting in Ryan's room or the airport this particular morning. My head was slightly dizzy and my heart was still throbbing. I typically welcome time on flights to read, but I did not have the focus or care for it that morning. I was finally facing reality: Ryan was going to be at school in Los Angeles and I was going to be working in Houston. And it was literally breaking my heart in two.

How It Started

I was taking in the view of the gorgeous rock formations and waterfalls at the Emerald Pools in Zion National Park. We were on spring break vacation in our last year of college with my parents, but on this hike we were alone. Ryan began saying something, but to be honest, my mind was completely absorbed in the serene landscape. The mountains were decorated perfectly with speckles of green foliage and the sun bounced gently off the still water in front of us. When he started talking broadly about our future life my ears took their cue and started to tune in. By the time I heard the words "will you marry me," he had my full attention. Although I was completely unprepared, I needed no time at all amidst my shock to immediately say, "YES!"

I did not expect a marriage proposal on this hike, which is exactly what Ryan wanted. This was three months before college graduation, and we had always said we were going to wait until after we finished college to get engaged. That being said, I was glad Ryan had found a way to surprise me. By this time, our lives were so intertwined and we knew each other so well, it could be hard to pull off a big surprise. But he had done it, and done it well!

Our paths intertwined freshman year of high school when we had all eight classes each day together. We went to the same school in our small hometown of Sparta, New Jersey, that boasted a whopping class size of about two hundred students from first through eighth grade, yet outside of that embarrassing stairwell incident in seventh grade, we had never met or spoken to each other. I knew of Ryan and that his dad was the wrestling coach, but Ryan did not even know my name, that is until freshman year when we saw each other constantly. We spoke a lot that year and by sophomore year we were dating. Then our paths crisscrossed until we made a knot and never looked back. Our old-soul personalities clicked, and I think we were both overjoyed to find a friend who was more interested in hiking the nature trail behind school than going to the secret party. We recognized the tendency to become overly competitive with each other, and I was secretly thrilled to learn his life dreams were just as ambitious as mine. With the first, we often ended up competing and with the second, we found a partner that believed in our dreams. It was clear to us and everyone around us that we were here to stay. As we got to know each other in that first year, we learned that although we understood each other so well, our childhoods could not have been more different.

Ryan's parents owned and operated a small plumbing business where they, by choice, selected jobs that were only in Sparta because they preferred not to travel. Years later, I would watch how this background in plumbing enabled Ryan to grow into an extremely effective engineer and scientist. My parents, by contrast, were both engineers who commuted almost an hour to work and traveled for their jobs. Especially my mom, who traveled extensively by the time Ryan and I met. When I was a freshman in high school she was offered the job of her dreams in France. As a teenager entering high school, moving to France when I did not speak French seemed devastating. All I wanted at that time was to fit in and be with my friends like any young teenager. I begged not to move to France and she accepted my wish and turned down the role. She always had, and I know always will, put me first and this was no exception. Her company did work with her to find a compromise and she ended up traveling to France half the time—two weeks there and two weeks home. Sometimes even traveling to other destinations in the two weeks she would have been home. This actually meant that Ryan did not meet her for a few months after we started dating because of her travel schedule. I know my father probably never wished she was home more than when he learned to navigate his daughter's new boyfriend coming over to the house (by the way, he did great!). And it was at our homes where we really saw how opposite our lives were. The first time Ryan ever came to my house, it was to deliver my homework after I missed a week of school from a terrible flu strain. He brought twelve roses for me and his smile was so bright. My grandparents happened to be visiting because it was my birthday and he won them over with his manners and charm. I would later learn how intimidated he was by the size of our house and meeting my family, something I had not even thought about.

The first time I went to Ryan's house, his mom greeted me at the door with a warm smile and reassurance that there was nothing to worry about, but his sister's snake had just gotten loose. She further explained it was not venomous, as she joined his sister and dad in their search . . . *but* I did still need to take my shoes off at the door. I quickly learned his household was much more active, with three siblings and two half-siblings in the mix, compared to mine as an only child, pretending my three cats were my siblings. A large family made up of mainly boys, Ryan's mom was always cooking meals, and in the summer, you could always rely on there being a delicious cake left on the counter in the afternoon. My family, on the other hand, always had dinner in restaurants. When we would drive around town, I would ask Ryan what he thought of different restaurants and was shocked each time he told me he had never been there. He, in turn, was shocked that I had been to all of them. This is probably where we had the most fun. As time passed, Ryan enjoyed exploring all the restaurants with my family and I loved eating his mom's homemade meals, experiences, which for both of us, had previously been rare treats. I particularly remember enjoying a mulligatawny soup and cornbread while we studied together once at his house.

Outside of eating, Ryan spent his evenings training for wrestling where his dad was the main coach. Ryan came from a long line of successful wrestlers and they took it seriously. I was pretty focused on athletics as well, mainly tennis, but I also took other lessons like art and piano. In fact Ryan would later tell me that when he first asked me on a date on weekdays, and I kept telling him which conflicts I had, he thought I was lying because I was not interested. It never even occurred to me that it would come across as fake because this had always been my life, but I now know that I was involved in an unusually high amount of activities. We were from different worlds. For some, these differences may have led to less ability to connect, but for us, it somehow drew us closer. We got to see another way to live life and we were ecstatic to get to participate in the other's world. There was so much to learn and discover beyond just ourselves. Our moms both became second mothers for us, and this opened new doors for each of us.

If there was a snow day or instance I needed a last minute ride, Ryan's mom stepped in, and when Ryan needed to go on a college visit or help with physics homework, my mom came to the rescue. There was a great synergy between our lives and both of our families filled a gap for us that we didn't know existed. Throughout all of this discovery, we got to know each other and see how, despite our divergent upbringings, when it came to ethics, morals, and enjoying life, we were extremely alike. It may seem crazy, and we knew we were young and drunk on love, but it was clear to us, by the end of our sophomore year in high school that one day, we would get married.

As it turns out, I had missed many signs that would have told me to expect the proposal on the hike. For weeks, Ryan had been telling me he felt this vacation was going to be extra special, but I would listen with half an ear as I made a checklist of everything we had to pack and never read into it. After he proposed, we laughed the whole way down the mountain as he finally got to tell me all the secrets he had been holding in that year and wanted to share with me. The stories were practically bubbling out of him like carbonation in a soda bottle; because I'm normally the one he would tell things to, it was excruciating not to be able to do so. For instance, he had asked to borrow my car numerous times to meet a teammate that lived off campus for a class project. What I didn't know was that he was borrowing my car to go to the jeweler for my ring. I had never questioned why he needed my car and always simply said yes to his request. He recounted how everyone kept telling him to stop telling them about the ring or plan while I was around several times throughout the year because I might hear and he was proud of how he knew it was safe to talk about it. He knew me well enough to know when I would listen. As we connected over the journey that led to that moment, I smiled at how deeply he knew me. All the stories portrayed such a caring and astute partner; Ryan knew how to tell when I was listening, when I wasn't—and most importantly, he knew I fully trusted him.

At the bottom of the mountain, we told my parents with nervous excitement. They were as unprepared as I had been, but once they recovered from their shock, they decided we had to celebrate at dinner. That night we celebrated *big*. In my memory, we ordered every appetizer, entree, and dessert on the menu. I do know for certain that we ordered a bottle of red wine. My family does not casually drink and may only have a drink once a year at a holiday gathering, if that, so this was a mark of a special occasion. We enjoyed everything that was ordered as we recounted distant and recent memories over our relationship. This really took us down memory lane since we had been together before either Ryan or I could legally drive.

The next day, we continued on with our vacation. Ryan and I climbed Angels Landing alone that morning because we had to leave Zion midday, which meant if we wanted to complete the hike, we needed to cut off an hour of time from the average four hours it takes most hikers. This added challenge fueled our innate ambition and sealed our resolve that we were going to get to the top. We took off with the vigor of speed walkers! When I looked around during the first two miles of the hike, there was gorgeous landscape on either side of us, not unlike any nice hike. We kept up our brisk walk while we soaked in the beauty of the salmon-colored sandstone all around us. As the mountain got steeper, we could see the famous switchbacks that looked like a zipper going straight up the mountain to hold it together. They cut back and forth across the mountain to make the hike more traversable where it rapidly gains altitude. Seeing these were so inspiring that our footsteps got faster. As we started winding our way around the switchbacks, I started to notice how crowded they were. We went from being alone to surrounded by people. The abrupt incline was slowing everyone down. Ryan and I both realized we were never going to make it back to my parents in time at this new pace. He looked back at me with determined eyes. "Do you want to see how fast we can do this hike? Let's run!" Perhaps against my better judgment I nodded and we were off to the races. I started running and the people we were passing became blurs in my periphery. Every few switchbacks I had to stop to catch my breath, and then I continued to run up the steep rock like a child trying to win a race against an adult decades older than them. With a fast-beating heart, I looked ahead to see a narrow spine of rock with chains drilled into it directly down the center. The path was only a few feet wide and when I looked over the cliff down to my right, my entire body instantly tingled with shivers. I would have had no way to gauge how far a distance down it was but I remembered reading it was just over 1,440 feet. I was in awe at the sight of this rock formation and simultaneously frightened. I was so grateful someone was brave enough to originally put these chains in to hold onto. I made sure one hand was always on a chain and I took one mindful step at a time. My confidence built as I came to see my footing was solid but I kept hearing a man behind. As I briefly glanced back, I saw a man's face, which was as red as Dorothy's slippers as if he had been holding his breath. He seemed to be really struggling and then I heard him pleading over how he is extremely afraid of heights. I couldn't fathom why he was up here and could only think that he needed to turn around. From the heavy, fast sound of his breath, I could tell he was almost in a full panic attack. I'm sure the many signs informing us that two to four people die on this hike a year and that you should use the chains were not helping. I felt for him and hearing his pleas of desperation made me realize that I was not the only one I needed to worry about. If anyone in this line slipped or made a drastic move out of fear, they could knock any of us right off this cliff! This made the trek scarier since many factors were out of my control. I observed everyone around me more closely as I kept putting one foot in front of the other over this potentially fatal ridge. When I took my last step out onto the summit, I let out a sigh of relief. Ryan and I walked out together onto the outlook and started looking around us mesmerized by the three-hundred-sixty degree view of a canyon all around us thousands of feet down with a backdrop of mountains. We had reached a pivotal summit in our lives that felt cheerful and exuberant. The other mountains in the distance could be seen as other peaks left to climb, but right then, I literally felt on top of the world. I'd never felt so alive. The view was simply magical. It truly cannot be described. Maybe not the most poetic or romantic of thoughts, but all I could say to myself was, *Life is good.* Just like those shirts and bumper stickers sold at every beach across America. I remember my mom telling me that day that I had not stopped smiling since Ryan proposed. I was floating in a sea of love. At least until the next morning. Sometimes I wish life, like Angels Landing, had chains you could hold on to when there is the potential danger of falling.

Ryan's face was sullen as he sat on the edge of the extra hotel bed looking at his computer. The amount of time he was looking at the screen and not looking up was concerning. "Is everything okay?" I asked him.

He looked up and soberly replied, "Just got an email that I didn't get into Rice University."

"What?!" I said. "But that is not possible." I walked over to see his computer screen. I read the email. I read it again. It was such a simple email and it confirmed what he had said. Again, I read the one sentence that would change our lives.

A dark cloud came over me. I went from my highest-high to my lowest-low in an instant. My heart was on the floor and tears were accumulating en masse as I fervently tried to hold them back. I tried to fathom how I was going to continue on with my day. We were going to the Grand Canyon with my parents in a few hours and at that moment it felt impossible to even move. Through this paralyzing, enveloping sadness, all I felt I could do was curl into a ball and cry. What was the point of even going to the Grand Canyon now anyway? That seemed so trivial when we had just learned our plans after graduation were over. We thought we had it all figured out: we were both going to move to Houston after graduation, live in warm weather, buy a nice house, and adopt a cat. We had worked hard for this and hard work pays off, right? Thoughts of denial slowly surfaced from my cloud of despair. *This has to be a mistake, we can fix this,* I thought. But was there truly a way to fix it?

We had been very fortunate up to this point in life. Out of high school, we were both accepted into Northwestern University and we had our sights set on ensuring we both found jobs in the same location after graduation. We had both completed many internships at companies across the country to try to increase the chances we had of getting a job in the same location, but our senior year, Ryan hesitantly mentioned to me that he may not actually want to go work in industry and instead pursue a PhD. Through his internships, he realized he needed a PhD to work on researching the cutting-edge technology that interested him. This was a big switch for someone to decide in their senior year of college. While most prospective PhD students had done as much research as possible in college, he had created a perfect resume for industry. I am not sure how many people could pull off switching to research so late in college (spoiler alert: he would pull this off successfully), but I have never doubted Ryan's ability. I made sure to tell him that I fully supported this change of plans because I, too, could sense that he had a passion for research and needed this to be happy long term. He was born to be a scientist and I was not going to stand in his way. The curveball in this was that I would have to accept a job offer in the fall and graduate school acceptances would not be announced until the following spring. This opened up a lot of unknowns and meant coordinating our careers would be much more difficult.

Immediately, we began planning for our postgraduation life, but unbeknownst to us, the Universe was doing some planning of its own. After spending five years surviving the brutal winters of Chicago, we were very over the cold weather. I refused to boil any more water to unfreeze my bike lock each morning, so this helped us narrow our search to Texas and southern California. We both applied to several places in both areas. By fall, after several months of interviewing, I had narrowed my options down to ExxonMobil in Houston and Chevron in Los Angeles.

In weighing these two choices, there was an internal motivation I had that added to the complexity of the decision: my dream was to live in California and train with the best yoga teachers in America. In college I had discovered yoga and I wanted to learn, understand, and know more, especially about how it can contribute to feeling calm and joyful. So, I was already leaning toward Chevron for the location. And let's be honest, California seemed like the place to be. Who doesn't want to see the sun all year round and have access to gorgeous beaches? After interviewing with them, I was even more convinced this was the location for me. My heart was ready to explore the West Coast and move to the multitude of high-quality yoga studios and sunny beaches of California!

To actually make the decision on where I would work, we weighed all the facts we knew. Keep in mind that the tasks of the jobs were almost identical, so the decision mainly came down to the benefits and location. And the more we listed those details, the more they pointed to Houston. Ryan had an almost guaranteed chance of getting into Rice so if we wanted to be together, the choice was Houston especially since ExxonMobil had a location in Los Angeles and Houston. My mom had come to the same conclusion when she looked at the financials and called to let us know her thoughts. "Hey, I compared the two offers as I said I would and wanted to let you know what I have come up with," she said.

"Okay, we have time now," Ryan replied. I asked my mom to review the offers, not only because of her extensive experience with engineering contracts from her career, but also because she was the person I'd always turned to during life's big transitions.

"Great. So this is really hard for me to tell you because, Sarah, I know you are really set on California, but I want to make sure you know the decision you are making. As we already knew, the ExxonMobil offer is better financially, but it was even more than I expected." She paused before proceeding to say it as gently as possible. "The ExxonMobil offer is a decent bit higher than Chevron to start and you have to account for no state income tax in Houston and 13 percent in California. Without taking into account anything else like cost of living, you are already looking at a wide gap. I know that probably sounds strange with a good salary, but California is just really expensive. You obviously have to choose what you want, but from a purely financial standpoint, Houston is your better option. I do think it will help you start your life out with a strong foundation," she explained.

Tears were slowly streaming down my face. The kind where your face is motionless, but a waterfall of tears is reflexively falling down your cheeks whether you want them to or not. A true silent cry. With every sentence another stream of tears surfaced. I was truly grateful to be in a place where I had this decision to make—the tears were not because I had to make this decision but because my heart wanted to set all the logic aside and choose the place that was calling my name. Yet I had only followed logic up to this point in my life and I sensed I would not have the courage to listen to my heart. I also recognized I had never gone to work to pay my bills or pay my rent full time, and I didn't want to make a bad decision from lack of experience based on a location I wanted to live in. It was important to me that I make sure I respected this privilege that was before me.

I honestly do not remember if I responded. I remember feeling almost frozen despite it being a toasty ninety-five degrees outside. Even with all the reasons hinting the opposite, my heart still wanted to choose Chevron. I had a deep craving I cannot explain to head to the West Coast, and I wanted to throw caution to the wind, but we had repeatedly decided if our main goal was to be together then I should choose the option that would most likely lead us there. And logically, that was clearly Houston. Loud and clear.

My body slightly trembled as I held my phone in my hand. I was procrastinating typing the number in because I didn't want to make the call. As I scanned the apartment, all I saw were beige walls and even beiger carpet. Ryan and I had just packed all of our stuff and loaded the car to go back to college from our fall internships in Houston. All that was left was the rented couch. The dreariness of the room matched how I felt. I often had trouble making decisions, but in this instance my heart was clearly speaking to me. There was an inner voice I had never heard before. Yet choosing California had the greater chance of separating Ryan and me, so I would choose Houston. One number at a time I finally pressed the Chevron recruiter's phone number and with each ring my blood pressure rose. As I told her my decision, I wished so much that she could know how much I appreciated this offer. That my expressed gratitude was not obligatory words to be professional. That in fact it was painful to turn down an offer I had wanted, but I needed to follow what was best for my personal life. When I hung up, a heaviness replaced the inner trembling and gentle tears started flowing. My heart and mind screamed, "No! No! No!" I looked up to see Ryan at the couch and I knew my path was now set. Now we just had to wait seven months to hear back from the universities to know if we would be together.

I accepted my ExxonMobil offer at the end of my internship. In the meantime, Ryan and I headed back to finish our senior year of college. We shoved the trunk shut with the car stuffed with our belongings and started the drive from Houston to Chicago. Every gas station exit for the next twenty hours of our trip would prove to have a large Chevron sign on the left and an equally large ExxonMobil sign on the right glaring down on us. I remember looking at Ryan six hours into the drive and saying, "The decision is already haunting me."

He looked back with a face that suggested I stop reading into signs, and said, "No, it is not. We made a decision. We chose what will most likely let us be together and we have a really good shot at that." I agreed. I was probably overreacting and reminded myself that I had chosen ExxonMobil because it gave us an almost guaranteed chance of being together, and I had really enjoyed my internships. But these signs were very real, and this decision would in fact prove to haunt me for many years.

Looking back, we were lucky to have plans to go to the Grand Canyon the day we heard back from Rice because it kept us from sinking too far into a canyon of our own despair. We would later learn his application was not even reviewed and he had received an automatic reply at the end of the admission season. It was probably possible for him to still get in, but begging for an application to be reviewed after the fact did not seem like a great way to start a PhD program. By this time, Ryan had been accepted into UCLA and had a fantastic experience while meeting the research group he would work with there. There was a team of about fifteen PhD candidates under the professor he applied for and he got to meet over half of them. He immediately got along with the other students and cared about the research they were conducting so he accepted their offer. He was going to be working in California, only a short drive away from where my heart told me to go in the first place.

Yes, it's true, I, too, could probably have called Chevron back and asked to work there, but burning bridges by revoking an accepted offer and fleeing to a competitor seemed like a less than optimal way to start my career. We had both worked really hard in college and both had big dreams. UCLA was clearly his best option and ExxonMobil mine. Neither of us wanted the other to sacrifice all they had worked for right from the start. Although it was an excruciating decision to make, we decided we would do long distance for a year until one of us could make a move that wasn't detrimental.

At *most* for a year.

Three

First Day

I found myself sitting at a restaurant with my new department head on my left, my supervisor across from her, and the rest of my team on my right. Just one week prior, Ryan and I had flown to Los Angeles to move him into his new place after he had helped me unpack in Houston. My cousin serendipitously lived in Houston and had graciously offered for me to move in with her family when she learned Ryan would not be joining me in Texas. I knew it would be supportive to return home to family instead of an empty house when just the past seven days had felt like a year. We had barely taken a step forward into this new life and many things had already triggered me, like the contract I had to sign stating that I would pay back my relocation fees if I left before two years of service. I knew 401(k) vesting was three years and pension eligibility was five years, but I wasn't ready for the relocation. I wasn't ready for a lot of what was to come. Every day brought something new. This particular day was my first day of work and I was at my welcome lunch.

We had already gone through all the basic formalities: roundtable introductions of name, role, where we grew up, and college attended. My department head glanced down to get something from her purse and she saw my hand. Her head lifted right back up as she looked at me and exclaimed, "Wow, what a lovely diamond you have! What does your fiancé do?" I wanted so desperately at that moment to pretend my sparkling stone was somehow not an engagement ring. I was lost for words. I wasn't prepared to say anything but the truth. "He is getting his PhD," I blurted wearily.

"Did he also come to Houston?"

"No, he is going to UCLA," I replied meekly.

"How long has he been in his program?"

"He started last week."

"Oh, so he just started a five-year program last week? Is it five years?"

Was there an invisibility cloak somewhere I could hide under? I wanted to melt right out of my seat. I had planned to avoid this subject as long as possible and here it was out in the open, curtains withdrawn, four hours into my job. My mom's stories of when she started engineering flooded back into my head. She was one of the only women then, and I recalled all the times she told me that she did not even mention having a boyfriend, and eventually husband, because promotions could be questioned if the company thought a woman may choose to have a child. Her friends had told me stories too, and I knew I may need to be cautious. There are more women in engineering now but it has traditionally been a male dominated field and some past biases still linger, like the belief that a woman will miss work if she has children or follow her husband's career. This leads to a culture where female employees keep parts of their personal life secret. You don't want to give any indication that you won't give 100 percent to your job or be willing to take on promotions. I was probably already on some employee watchlist of people likely to leave the company. How was I going to be seen as serious? I typically operate as an open book, but I was quickly sensing that it was time to take my heart off my sleeve and tuck it away somewhere safer.

My heart couldn't handle any more aches.

Four

Sundays

The first time I flew between Houston and Los Angeles, I took note of the time I left my door and entered Ryan's door. It was an eight-hour journey. Even more if you included the time zone change. That is how I counted the space between us. In my mind, there was a gap defined by time. And that time was defined by technology. To get to him required driving a car to the airport, riding the parking shuttle to the terminal, flying on a plane, waiting for an Uber, and finally taking an Uber to his door. This gap seemed far too large and it certainly added to my agitation. Up to that point, I had only been thinking about the flight. I had calibrated to a three-and-a-half-hour flight, but I had missed that it was really a seven-to-ten-hour trip depending on wait times between each mode of transit. I wanted to complain loudly and repeatedly about how this was completely unfair. Like a child throwing a tantrum and the parents make sure to right the wrong. My hope being that by some miraculous stroke of luck someone would hear and it would change the distance between us, but I knew the situation wasn't changing anytime soon. We had made this decision and it was just the beginning. I shook off the thought of this being too long and looked forward. This was called a *long*-distance relationship after all.

We decided to visit each other once a month. We would alternate who flew to who each month. In the beginning, Ryan was still taking classes which made it harder for him to fly to me because he had to take Friday off or he would spend all day Saturday flying with the time change. At the same time, I was on call twenty-four seven with my job. In order to leave, I had to get a backfill. This meant I had to find someone in the company who was trained to do my job and who was willing to take my phone calls while I was out of town. This always left me with a feeling of guilt. When I asked someone to backfill, I felt like I was saying, "Hi, can you please potentially ruin your weekend by being ready to do my job so I can go visit my fiancé?" There could not be any spontaneous flights or road trips because I needed to give others advance notice. This was a part of my new job that I had to learn to manage, and it made me feel like the distance between us was even greater. We maneuvered all these details out of necessity, but I really felt the strain of our hectic schedules and flying.

Fortunately, we also learned a major upside of long distance: every visit is like a mini honeymoon. You drop everything going on in your life and completely enjoy the thirty-six to forty-eight hours you have with each other. When I picked Ryan up from the airport, I would always run out of my car to give him a hug. I would be in disbelief that he was really there. The moment had finally come for us to be together again. I recall all these memories of our first hug after a month apart fondly—me running up and finally feeling his warmth in a big cozy embrace—but Ryan recalls that people were not happy we were holding up traffic. I know our ten-second hugs did not cause any backlog of cars, but Ryan was always conscientious of the vehicle parked behind us. To this day, he describes these encounters with people honking and cursing at us to move forward. It is one of his superpowers to be aware of how everyone feels around him, and sometimes I have to remind him that it is okay to take a few seconds. They will be okay, we won't even change their day.

These honeymoons together became vacation sprints. We were living in two big cities and had a lot to explore. We became tourists in each other's city while acting like locals. Over many trips, there were more adventures than I can remember. In Houston, we visited NASA and got a personal tour because my cousin's husband worked there at the time. We also went to Galveston to see Moody Gardens and the beach with her family. Ryan and I explored downtown by walking Memorial and Buffalo Bayou Park as well as going to several of the most popular restaurants. Uchi may still be at the top of our recommendation list. In Los Angeles, I always requested to go to a beach. We walked the serene and often busy sands of many beaches with friends . . . Venice, Dockweiler, Santa Monica. The beach we frequented most often was Santa Monica because an incredible donut shop called Sidecar Doughnuts is close by. Donuts are not typically my dessert of choice, but my favorite part of these Saturday morning trips was that Ryan and his roommates truly did frequent this shop often, and I got to share in one of their regular activities. I would be so happy as I ate my Thai-tea flavored donut, sipped my matcha latte, and listened to everyone laughing. I would be filled with gratitude for the moment and simultaneously filled with sadness because I could not always join them. That is the ultimate paradox of long distance. You get to have two homes, explore two places, and meet twice as many friends, but you only get to share memories occasionally when you are visiting. Luckily, this makes you treasure the opportunities you get, and we did see more of LA than just a donut shop. We visited the Getty Villa, Hollywood Walk of Fame, Universal Studios, Los Angeles County Museum of Art, Huntington Library, and La Brea Tar Pits to name just a few. Being a tourist without paying for a hotel and rental car really is a plus . . . long distance is in no way easy so you really have to look at the positives that are part of the journey.

We had the best time exploring the areas we now called home, but when Sunday evening came we started to feel like we had not really seen each other. The entire weekend would be filled with plans since we had such a short time. We both met new friends in our cities and naturally they always wanted to meet our partner when they were in town. But it became too much. We needed some alone time, so we shifted our weekends. Every honeymoon, we set aside at least four hours, if not a half day, where it would only be the two of us. This drastically improved the quality of our visits. Occasionally, we even reserved a full weekend where we were completely alone. Some of the best times we had were mini-weekend trips. In Texas, we separately visited Austin, San Antonio, and Fort Worth. Austin was a mini-weekend trip we were not prepared for! We showed up Saturday to a warm, eighty-degree day and we hiked all day in the warmth and sunshine. The next morning, we stepped outside to find Sunday was a chill, twenty-eight degrees. Suddenly we weren't hiking but shopping for winter coats and spending time staying warm inside the flagship Whole Foods Market, which I am still awed by to this day. Each trip, just like the Austin one, had its own quirks, and I will always cherish these Texan memories. We did also do some weekend trips in LA, but as Ryan did not have a car there, these were always with friends. The one I enjoyed the most was sharing a house with eight friends on Catalina Island. It was a spectacular weekend, but I must admit that it felt strange getting off the ferry and I was the only one who needed to catch a ride to the airport. It was these moments where the feeling of loneliness and separation would set in.

The Sundays we had to fly home were the hardest for me. I would get extremely sad. Typically tears would surface against my wish. I always seemed to take it harder than Ryan. I would feel like my reaction was quite drastic and he was calm. One day I asked him, "Aren't you sad?" I did not understand how he just accepted that it was already time to part after seeing each other for only one full day. "Of course I am," he said, "I just react differently." On some level I accepted this answer. I should have realized we all handle situations differently. His sadness may just not express itself in tears. Maybe he was holding it all in or maybe he reacted when I was not around. On another level, I did not accept his answer. I did not want to be the only one who appeared to struggle on Sundays. I think I knew I was not able to process my emotions fully and was hoping he would show some sign of weakness. It is hard to admit, but I was trying to pull Ryan down to my level. Then I could justify my behavior. I saw myself sinking and did not want to sink alone. I really was asking, "Will you join me in my craziness?" This would have allowed me to not face my obstacle. Luckily, Ryan did not cave to my hidden request.

I had many Sundays to learn how to grow. With each one I would get to face my darkness again until I could shift my perspective. Each trip started and ended with a hug; one marked by overflowing joy and the next marred by inescapable sadness. Sometimes the weekends were so short that it felt like a tease. Your best friend was there just for a second. When I got really sad and Ryan was flying home, he would always say, "I have to go back so I can graduate and we can be together. I am working really hard so I can graduate as fast as I possibly can." I heard those words many times and tried to imagine what that day would look like, but it always felt so far away. I truly had trouble visualizing that the day would come. When I had to fly home, it always felt like a strange déjà vu. Everything felt familiar and foreign as all the steps I had just taken to arrive were spun in reverse. I walked back into the airport and went to my gate often to find it was the same gate I left from. Across from the gate would be a Peet's Coffee that I had gotten tea from two days before. Despite the short time span, my mind felt like it must have been over a week ago. Simultaneously, when I would see the various parts of the airport it would suddenly feel like I was just there hours ago—traveling like we were doing really made time feel like it had expanded. On top of that, it was like my nervous system was frozen from the pain which caused time to warp in either direction. Once the plane landed, I walked through the same Houston terminal halls to the parking shuttle, handed them my slip with my car location, and waited patiently on the shuttle as I was inevitably dropped off last. When I arrived back home, the air felt stale. The sting of loss was so fresh as I was acutely aware that Ryan was not there. I'd scan the living room, all of my belongings would be right where I left them. I'd see a to-do list on the kitchen table, a stack of books on the chakras that I was studying, or a recently purchased pack of lightbulbs for a light that went out. Each item would slowly remind me of my life and the week ahead. I'd start to question what we were doing and why we only got brief moments together. These reflections would often be very late at night because we would book the latest flight home possible to maximize our time together. This made for some very difficult Mondays. I struggled through those work days with a generous amount of black tea, but the responsibility of work the next day would restart my routine. I would fall back into my usual pattern and remember why I had to return. I had a job and a full life in Houston that I was living. In just a day or two, I would be back in the swing trying to recall what it was like seeing Ryan just a short time ago. It was eerie how easy it was to readjust to being apart. One night you can't imagine being apart and another you can't imagine what it would be like to live together. I never got over that. The shift happened every time—month after month. It was an emotional roller coaster.

Forget. Remember. Repeat.

Five

A Year

My mom was visiting me sometime in our first year apart. She has always visited me everywhere I have lived and is my biggest supporter. My whole life she has been the main person encouraging me to work hard, live my dreams, and believe anything is possible. She is unbelievably dedicated to everything she does and, as my mom, she would answer the phone for me any time of day no matter where she is in the world. In fact, she has answered the phone in the middle of the night for me several times.

On this day, we were casually talking as we drove from my place to a restaurant. We hit some minor traffic as I was driving, and she asked me how work was going. I mentioned something about it only being for a year, so there was only so much impact I could make. I had made it a point to mention that this situation was only going to be for a year, many times over the last few months.

"You know, Sarah, this could turn into more than a year. It could be possible that you are here for two years," my mom stated matter of factly.

"I don't want to talk about that," I snapped harshly as I maneuvered us through the traffic. I knew I had not answered kindly, but my pain was too great for me to rationally discuss what might happen if this life lingered longer than a year. Limiting our time apart to one year was my armor of protection. It helped me get through each day, knowing we were closer to bridging the space between us. This was obviously a form of denial and I, along with everyone else, could see that. I know my mom was just helping me nudge closer to reality, probably concerned that I could be hurt further if my delusional bubble burst unexpectedly, but I was too emotionally torn apart to go there. I also knew my mom felt I was angry at her for encouraging me to go to Houston. This was really hurting her since all she wanted was to support me and see me happy. The truth was I was not really angry at her; I was angry at the world. I did not know where to direct my emotions, so I just became angry at everything and everyone.

Seeing that it would take time for me to own that I was in Houston, my mom offered me one piece of advice that day in the car. She asked me to try not to hold resentment toward Ryan. She knew how easy it is to resent a life circumstance when we are angry and really didn't want me to hurt the special relationship that Ryan and I have. I did listen here and despite all my anger and disappointment, I really did make sure to let go of any resentment toward Ryan that tried to surface. I just didn't always apply that principle toward myself. Letting go of how I wanted my life to be was harder. I had believed that I could create the life I wanted, and I had worked really hard to land in a place I had not imagined and quite frankly didn't love. This was one of the first times I was forced to open up to the possibility that something bigger beyond my vision was trying to happen.

Maybe I was getting exactly what I needed instead of what I wanted.

Six

Type A

"How are you and Ryan doing? Is he enjoying his program?" my supervisor asked me. I assured her we were well and then answered the other questions that were as close as possible to asking if I was going to leave the company without asking. I knew it was her job to be nosy while staying politically correct. I, in turn, did my job to confidently affirm that I was not going anywhere and everything was great. When we completed this obligatory dance, we were able to talk about my work. A little ways into our conversation she broke out into a soft laughter and proclaimed, "It is so nice to have someone here who is not the typical Exxon type A personality! We really do need people like you to bring a new perspective and uplifted energy to the office." She truly meant this in the best way but I did not interpret it that way. I knew not being seen as type A would be negative for me in performance reviews. The company was well known for ranking every employee and where you landed in the list of 70,000 employees determined your raises and promotions. This created a very competitive environment and I thought I had proven I was competitive and ambitious. Which is true, I am. But I wasn't perceived as this or I didn't check the other boxes of type A, I guess. I could put that aside, but what I really heard was that I did not fit in, and that really bothered me. I felt like the ugly duckling who everyone could see was different and didn't know why. Since my first day of work, I had been hiding parts of myself, knowing that I often didn't meet the status quo of the culture. I had learned to not wear my colorful, free spirited blouses and to stick more with neutrals or better yet the company FRC (Fire Retardant Clothing) uniforms that were mandatory in the field. I also did my best not to get into a conversation that revealed I was vegetarian; that was like sinning in Texas. It consumed my energy and now I was hearing that I needed to cover up even more if I wanted to be viewed like my peers. I knew realistically this was never going to happen, so I felt like I was sent to an island by myself.

My friend Lorena was the one person I could count on at work to truly understand me. When I walked into the visitor center on my first day of work, the first person I saw was Lorena. I couldn't believe it. We had not seen each other in over two years. She walked toward me with the same vibrancy I remembered. Her heart was held high, there was a sparkle in her eye, and she walked with a bouncy confidence that she was headed somewhere. Even more petite than me, at five feet, Lorena's energy radiated in a way that let the world know she was very capable. Plus, she was always dressed to the T with her long black hair perfectly blown dry. I've always been in awe that she could work out in the morning and get to work with perfect hair and makeup. "Lorena!" I called.

"Sarah! Oh my gosh, hi, how are you? Is this your first day too?" I was ecstatic to see someone I knew. We discovered that it was both of our first days and we would both be in the chemical plant. After this short exchange, her supervisor arrived to bring her upstairs so we said goodbye and that we would catch up later as I waited for mine to arrive.

Type A

Lorena and I had met at ExxonMobil while working as interns three years prior. We became good friends during that time, but had not kept up with each other much afterward. A year later we discovered that we were both interning in San Francisco for different companies. Naturally, we decided we had to meet up in the city for lunch. There are so many restaurants in San Francisco that it was hard to choose one, but we landed on a vegan upscale Mexican restaurant for lunch. It was quite memorable with its adobe architecture and flavorful meals. Looking back now, it really reflected our personalities in many ways. While there, we picked up right where we had left off like no time had elapsed. After we left San Francisco, we again did not keep in touch and had not talked until seeing each other in the visitor center.

Shortly after Lorena left, my supervisor arrived to show me up to my office. We walked down a hall I was familiar with from my days as an intern. It was one of those places where the interior was still stuck in the seventies. The walls between offices were textured vinyl and many of the chairs were the orange lounge chairs where the arm rest is wood with a strip of padded orange fabric on top. The outside of the building was all glass and the only part that had aged well. The whole thing had been top of the line, at some point. My supervisor stopped at a door half way down the hall. "This will be your office and here is your key," she announced as she pointed to a door. I looked up and saw my name neatly printed on a nameplate. I looked to my right and was shocked to see Lorena's name neatly printed on the nameplate next to mine. Our lives were serendipitously intersecting again for the third time. This time we would stay in touch and see each other for more than three months as we had during our internships together. Lorena would become a close friend, maybe more aptly described as my work wife, as I would come to call her. We helped each other navigate this large organization we had just joined. We would go to each other for advice about the new hire training or comfort the other when there had been a difficult meeting. We were there for each other. Lorena was a huge supporter of me in my first year in Houston. She made the days less lonely, and I could feel how she fully accepted me. I could share my spiritual yoga journey with her without judgment and I could feel that she really understood me. This outlet where someone saw me for who I was and didn't want to change me, truly helped me make it through some difficult days in a culture where I normally didn't feel I belonged.

I recall so many moments that emotionally built up day after day. I walked into the control center one afternoon and heard an operator suddenly saying, "SHH, SHH, SHHHHH! No more cussing, there's a lady present." Everyone immediately listened and stopped the previous conversation. I wondered what they were talking about and if they perceived me walking in as interrupting their fun. I didn't want this politeness. I wanted to be treated equally, but that wasn't going to happen when I had already been quickly labeled a Yankee for being from New Jersey and someone who may think I am better than others since I went to a distinguished college.

One day my operations lead called me over. "Sarah, come to the parking lot with me. I have something to show you." I followed him out to the parking lot and he told me to look out at the vehicles and tell him what I saw. First was my light blue Ford Fusion Hybrid, and, then next to it, ten or more Ford F-150 trucks all painted in neutrals. At least I had the Ford part correct? I knew exactly what he was going to say. Once I had enough time to scan the lot, he told me that if I was going to work here, I needed to buy a new vehicle. This car was not going to cut it and he wanted to help me, but unlike my supervisor's attempt at a compliment, his was a disguised judgment. It stung to know I was not respected because I did not blend in. I was not about to buy another vehicle, let alone a truck, and I knew this meant I would have to work extra hard to gain respect for my work. It was tiring to be misunderstood, day in and day out, and feel I could not be my authentic self. It added to my feeling of loneliness from moving away from Ryan. I walked back to the control center solemnly wondering how I was going to navigate this environment. How would I connect and could it be done without straying further from myself?

Just as I shut the door, I heard the word *shit* and then another frantic directive to hush echo around the room.

Seven

Criticism

I quickly learned the pull of social expectations for a couple in a long-distance relationship is great. The barrage of criticisms we received for remaining long distance truly surprised me. I could see people did not even realize how much they were being led by groupthink whenever the conversation came up. When did everyone decide there is only one way to live? I was subjected to so many comments every day—

"Why would you choose long distance?"

"Oh, is your husband in the military?"

"I cannot imagine doing what you are doing."

"And you trust him being out in LA by himself?"

The most common comment I continually received when they found out Ryan and I were living apart was, "Oh, you must be so lonely!" How do you answer a comment like that? Yes, thank you for the reminder! It's not exactly the easiest question to answer, especially when you are insanely lonely. I'd normally mutter something undefinable, or quip a short "I'm alright" because I realized very quickly that no one wants to hear that you really *are* lonely, and I didn't want to talk about it anymore than they did. Being reminded always hurt, especially if the person really didn't understand how I was feeling. These fleeting remarks forced me to admit that although I was surrounded by people, it was true that I felt alone. And to me, I think there may be no worse feeling than being pitied by another person. Pity communicates the message, "I think you are small and maybe weak enough to need saving." I may have felt broken but I was not weak, and did not want to be treated as such.

Most comments I could normally let slip by since they did not know me and we had little to no connection. It was the judgements from our close family and friends which hurt the most. I never imagined they would contribute or even have an opinion. I naively assumed they would respect our decision and at least outwardly show support.

"Why would you do that?"

"Are you sure about long distance, life is really short?"

"Will you get a new job?" One day Ryan was with me when this question was asked. As we walked away, he said with a heavy heart, "I don't like how you are the only one who was looked at when that question was asked."

"Yeah, I know, I noticed it too. I'm never asked if you will get a new job."

"I'm sorry, babe. You know I don't just expect that you'll follow me right? We'll talk about it when we get there," he replied.

"I know. Thanks. Unfortunately, I still have to answer this question constantly." For as long as we were apart, this question was directed at me. Even when Ryan and I were standing together, physically in a room, their eyes would fix directly on me as they asked the question that was really none of their business. Women are still expected to follow their husband's career and give up on theirs, whether or not they have children.

"I would be so lost. I wouldn't be able to last a week," people would say.

"Do you have concerns about fighting when you eventually share a place again?"

"Are you going to delay the wedding?" No. NO. NOOOO! I wanted to scream!

Honestly, it had never even crossed my mind to delay or cancel the wedding until people started asking if we were. Why would we do that when our love for each other had not changed? Just our locations. I knew true love could make it through anything. What we had was genuine, and no obstacle would prevent us from shining. Internally, I was clear on this, and it was the only question I knew how to answer. Unfortunately, I was still grappling with being apart which allowed most of the comments to build up inside me. People who barely even knew me seemed to care deeply enough about this pivot from social norms to provide their own input. Why did so many strangers feel the need to comment or provide advice? Why did they care how I lived? Did they even realize that stating their opinions out loud was hurtful? I'm pretty sure they did not realize this because of how fast their responses were. There was no time for reflection or filtering thoughts—it was pure reflex.

I've reflected on these questions and wondered why everyone seemed to care. Some things I will never know but I suspect it was a combination of reasons. Ryan and I had been together since we were just kids and those who knew us, saw us as a pair. People loved seeing us together and it was almost like we reinvented reality, splitting off into the incorrect parallel universe by going our own separate ways. Part of this pain, I very much felt myself. This feeling was reinforced by the fact that our situation was repairable. I could have quit my job and gotten another or Ryan could have reapplied to different graduate programs. There is a lot more leniency and respect for couples in positions where they do not have control of living together such as being in the military or a Secret Service position. I do feel a lot of the judgment came from us choosing to live out where we had landed. I get why people didn't understand our choice, but one thing about me is that I don't make decisions solely based on what I want; I try to make decisions based on what best serves my life and those around me in the long run. I've always been more focused on the long-term strategy than instant gratification, and in this case, running back to Ryan was not going to support my career or anyone else for that matter and changing schools for Ryan would have been a huge disadvantage.

I was not sure if I would regret this decision or if I was going to get a different job to be together after a few months. I took it day by day, but I could not let go of the fact that I had not followed my heart to accept the Chevron offer that would have brought me to California, and California was where Ryan now was. As much as I tried, and boy, did I *try*, I could not accept the choice I had made and it made me very angry, mostly with myself. But I didn't know what to do with it, how to process the anger. In fact, the anger became so pervasive that even hearing "Los Angeles" on the news became a trigger word for me.

It took me a while to recognize that I was in the midst of my first heartbreak. I didn't understand why it was so painful because our relationship had not ended, we were still very much together. I was questioning my decision and that was hard enough. I did not need other people's unsolicited feedback when I was still reconciling how I had not listened to my inner voice and ended up apart from Ryan. Each comment added salt to my oozing wound because each comment seemed to imply to me that people assumed we were exactly where we wanted to be, as if we were living our ideal lives. This of course was not ideal.

There are only two circumstances, excluding those involving my parents, I can remember when people responded supportively. These words are etched into my mind because they were in such stark contrast to all the others I heard everyday. An elderly lady sitting on the plane next to me who was traveling with her granddaughter from Los Angeles going back to Houston was making small talk, as you do when getting settled on a plane. After we got our seatbelts on she asked why I was headed to Houston. I felt myself tense up, and then decided to be honest. After all, I was never going to see this lady again. I explained our situation, and was shocked to see kindness reflected in her eyes when she said, "Oh, that is so wonderful. You both are really putting your future first and setting yourselves up for success. You are very wise to do that. I know that must be hard now. You will be happy you did this one day." She then promptly helped her young granddaughter straighten her Minnie Mouse ears from Disneyland. I sat quietly in surprise and felt invigorated by her words of encouragement. It only takes a little positivity to bolster someone up. As I tucked into my book as we got ready to take off, I thought about how lucky her granddaughter was to have such a forward thinking grandma to look up to in her life.

The second time was when I told my future yoga teacher about my situation. Without hesitation she responded, "That shows you have a strong character." I will always remember those words. They were words I really needed to hear at that moment. They reminded me that although this journey was difficult, it could be worthwhile.

Those comments from a stranger and my yoga teacher taught me that there were people present in my life who could see beyond the invisible fences of societal constructs. I'd be lying if I didn't admit how much I needed that reassurance.

I knew the answers to the questions I received every day about how my story was going to end, as much as the person asking them. It took me time to learn how to answer the questions that were often cloaked in criticisms. A lot of my energy was consumed by the emotions these conversations brought up and thinking about how to answer before I really got intentional about how I approached the daily inquiries. I started to provide very short responses, or I would be honest and say that I would rather not talk about it. At work, I had a one line answer prepared and kept it on repeat: "We are long distance right now while Ryan completes his PhD and then he will find a job in Houston." My mom, in particular, mentored me on how to handle the questioning at work. Have my story. Repeat it. Move on. While all of this was depleting and exhausting, looking back, I can see now that I needed to learn boundaries. I didn't owe anyone an explanation.

If I wanted to pour my heart out to a close friend and speak deeply, then I could. If I wanted to stop the conversation right after the question, then I could. I did not need to hear how they did not approve of my lifestyle choices when my response did not meet their preconceived notions. They weren't going to understand my journey, but most importantly, I didn't need them to. This was my life and I was not responsible for making others feel comfortable by providing a response that they condoned. As a lifelong emotional mediator, this was a powerful new way to live for me. It felt uncomfortable at first, so I naturally slipped in and out of remembering that I did not owe anyone an explanation because I was not responsible for the feelings of others. I slowly got stronger at not adding justifications to each passing comment, or more aptly judgment, and when I succeeded, I started to clearly see I had value regardless of my choices and how they were perceived. My worth was not connected to whether I lived under the same roof as my fiancé, lived the way others preferred, or lived by justifying my every move. I could choose how to be and approve of this myself. The only person who needed to know why I had made a decision and approve of that decision was me, and that is where I still had work to do. I was angry with myself for not listening to my intuition and this is another reason I probably received, or felt I received, so much criticism. I was sensitive to every word people said and therefore I heard all of it amplified. Where I normally would have brushed off a comment or not even paid attention, I would take every sentence in as another reminder that I had taken a different path than my heart had wanted. My pain was raw and every word cut into my mind with more meaning because I was not confident in my choice.

I was not clear yet. In many ways, I still felt like a victim instead of a strong individual who had made the best decision I could with the information that I had.

With each passing comment, another crack formed in my emotional shell. With each passing judgment, I neared closer to shattering.

Eight
Phone Calls

Ryan and I discovered that finding time to talk was one of the hardest parts for us in this new arrangement. The time zone difference was only two hours, but it significantly impacted weekdays. When I left for work, it was 5:30 a.m. for Ryan, so he was still sleeping. When Ryan got home at night, it was normally already 9:00 p.m. my time, so we had about one hour of the day where we were both free to talk. This was better than nothing, but being on my phone right before sleeping was not an ideal bedtime routine and Ryan typically needed to make dinner after a long day. This combination led us to not speak by phone very often. We did text everyday and this is how we kept up with what the other was doing. However, after some time went by, we soon came to realize that we rarely spoke by phone. I remember my frustration reaching a tipping point a few months in and declaring that we needed to talk more. We both agreed we would try to do better. This tipping point turned out to not move the needle and we ultimately had to schedule two times a week to talk. We are not people who really enjoy chatting on the phone a lot to begin with and, coupled with the time change, we found structure was required.

When people asked how often we spoke, they were often surprised by how infrequently we called each other. Sometimes they were even appalled. I always found it interesting that they would have a genuine reaction to how often we chose to talk. I did not see how it affected them. I was really never sure why there was an expectation to talk every day. That always seemed suffocating to me. How could you do the activities you wanted to after work each evening if you were always on the phone? In any case, we found the rhythm of what worked for us and there was more for us to learn.

"I just can't keep listening to this every time we talk, Sarah," Ryan said firmly. My mind searched frantically for what I said that would lead him to say this.

"What do you mean?"

"It just always sounds like your life is falling apart these days," he replied.

I was confused, because it kind of was. What else was I going to provide updates on? I felt it was important to share what I was going through with Ryan and I was simply explaining the present moment. It was true that I had much to be happy about as well. I was grateful that I had found my dream yoga school, but I was barely making it through each day and that was drowning out a large chunk of the good. I couldn't even eat dinner anymore because I had developed this intense heartburn. I was feeling both the happiest and saddest I had ever felt at the same time.

When I explained this, Ryan empathized but continued to insist he needed to hear more about the good. Since our time on the phone was so short, we often only got through the negative updates. I did understand his perspective, but I really felt I needed to be able to share what I was going through with him. Ever since I was fifteen years old I could easily talk to Ryan anytime I wanted. Suddenly, we barely had any time to talk and I was feeling the effects of not being able to share and process my emotions. My stories were building inside of me, most notably in the form of a faint heartburn, and their normal outlet was not there. I needed a solution that didn't involve only sharing my gratitude list and pretending everything was rainbows and sunshine.

If you had asked me before we were long distance how healthy our relationship was, I would have replied with heartfelt honesty, *very*. We almost never fought. We had the usual bickering, but it was mostly just teasing each other. In high school, we realized that our lives had collapsed on each other too much. All of our classes were the same, we spent every second possible together, and people often viewed us as one person. I later learned that there is an actual term for this called *codependency*, which the Oxford Learner's Dictionary defines as "a situation in which two people have a close relationship in which they rely too much on each other emotionally, especially when one person is caring for the other one." We did rely on each other emotionally and I did often seek approval. We put effort into repairing this in college. With different majors, we finally were in different classes, we got our own hobbies, and if friends texted only one of us about plans, we made it clear that we both needed to be texted. We also did several spurts of time apart in college for internships and none of this raised any problems. These shorter experiences apart showed us that we could live independently. I don't want to undermine our progress in these years, but our new, more uncertain long-distance relationship was showing me where there still was more work to be done. When you grow up side by side with someone since you were fifteen years old, there can be a lot to unravel as you become adults. There were still codependent ties remaining. I hadn't realized how much the little interactions Ryan and I had each day eased my stress. It felt like an emotional blanket was instantly gone when we went our separate ways. I was used to getting hugs multiple times a day. I was used to him coming up to me while I read to softly kiss my forehead. I was used to holding hands as we walked to town. These moments had made a significant difference to my days and they couldn't be replicated by phone. I now know, through yoga, that these moments were coregulating our nervous systems, which can also be healthy as long as you're not dependent on it, but I didn't have the words then to know what I was experiencing. I just knew that there was a feeling of deep unease that resided when the moments were gone.

Ryan, a natural problem solver, came up with a solution to ensure he could hear more than just my woes. He asked me to write him a letter and said I could write him as long as I wanted. As if to make sure I would agree with this idea, he added to send it in the mail. I felt pretty significant hesitation, but I was willing to try for Ryan and he had offered a solution for me to tell him what was happening after all. I got out a notebook. I had no idea where to start, so I just started to write . . .

> *Ry,*
>
> *I am going to just write this stream of consciousness. It would take me forever to organize the months of thoughts I have had. I do not know where to start, but I know I am not okay yet better than ever too. I am learning I am stronger than I knew. However, I also feel I have been broken. My core is not grounded from all the shattering that is happening. Work and Padma give feedback that I need increased confidence. This personality gap is screaming at me from all angles of life. So now I have to rebuild and then exceed any level of confidence and presence that I had before. I want this distance over but I know I am not meant to leave here yet. I may sound crazy, but I feel I am*

here to learn to trust the process of life, develop a stronger core, and learn what love means. Without being apart, I would have never spent so much time learning about deep trust and that everything happens for me.

One of my biggest heartaches with being separate and us struggling to make the phone work is not getting to express my dreams for the future and planning with you. I feel a deep desire to talk with you and reflect but I have not because I do not think you have the time and I respect that you're going through as much change as me. This desire is building up inside. We are living in two different worlds. You are still in school and swamped with homework, research, and finding out where you'll steer your career. And I'm onto working full time which is . . . well, you'll be right here until you're sixty years old if you don't dream. These first few years have caused so much reflection. I can see how it can easily turn into years of living the same day over and over until another holiday season or spring break passes by. It makes me reflect on whether it is CEO or marketing or leaving the industry completely that I am seeking. My visions of what is possible come faster than they can manifest—a blessing and a curse. A part of me has too little patience and another part of me never wants to discover I did not do today what I need to obtain the best later down the road. My biggest fear deep down may be that I will die without having changed the world. I fear I will not have the courage to leave industry and open a yoga studio. I fear there is even something much bigger than a studio I could do that I'll miss. I fear I will miss this from a fear of failure, and I do not know if I can be selfless enough to reach my full potential. I see that leaving the world a

> *better place means true dedication in every moment and not always choosing comfort or luxury . . .*

I kept writing—I wrote a *long* letter. I looked down at all the words on the pages. It was a raw, unedited novel of my emotional landscape. I no longer had any desire to send this to Ryan. He didn't need to know all of this information. This wasn't about him needing to know, this was about me needing to know, and then getting it out of me. I continued to write many more times after this first night. Free writing in my journal often revealed beliefs or thoughts I was harboring that I wasn't aware of. It created a pathway which brought these to the surface so I could look at them and decide if they were really true or helpful on my own. This process also freed up a lot of time for Ryan and I to talk about whatever we wanted. Phone calls improved, and we were both better off for it.

I learned journaling is a magical medium that day.

Nine

Failure

Amidst wedding planning, a new job, and learning to live outside the confines of school—this is where my ambitious attitude shined—I had added to my plate and signed up for a yoga teacher training course at a studio called Rasa Yoga School. Asana Immersion was an all-weekend workshop that went late Friday and had an early morning start both Saturday and Sunday for three consecutive weekends. The Sanskrit word *asana* translates to *posture* so this was the workshop to learn postural alignment and energetics. I started the workshop and found myself struggling to make it through the first Saturday afternoon. I was loving the material, and eager to learn, but could barely focus because I was so tired. My head hurt. Everything felt a bit hazy. My shell had cracked. Sunday morning I woke up, and as I struggled to make my eyes focus and lift my head off the pillow, it was clear that I was not going to be able to train for another full day. I threw my head back on the pillow, heavy with the realization that I wanted so badly to finish this training, but I simply wasn't physically capable. Then a small rush of panic ran over me when I realized the worst part: we had all left our mats in their respective spots the day before because we were going to be returning the next morning. Everyone would see my spot was empty and realize I had failed. It was just another thing to add to the moments where I would not meet others' expectations or receive the approval I so wanted. Feeling desperate to find a way to ground myself, I drove to the studio and tucked into the back of my favorite morning class. It had started later than the early workshop began, so I felt pretty sure no one would see me. When class was through, I tried to occupy myself with locating my keys when I saw my mentor Gracie coming toward me.

"I'm surprised to see you taking another class this morning, Sarah . . ." was all she said. My cheeks flushed as I searched for an appropriate answer. She accurately sensed my current state of overwhelm and exhaustion, and pulled me aside for a more private conversation. With her entire attention focused on what I was saying, I found I couldn't talk without tears flooding my face. I didn't want to cry, but I had no more strength to pretend I was strong. I told her what was going on with work, wedding planning, and my health through sniffles and sobs. I let it all pour out of me and then I explained to her that it had been so hard to focus all weekend after such demanding work weeks, and how my lack of sleep left me without any resilience to manage the stern talking-tos I was receiving at work. My work environment was harsh and even though yoga training wasn't per se, even being told to hold poses for long stretches was more than I could take. Everything was too hard. She spoke with me for a while and I vividly remember her saying, "One thing you can reflect on is what level of presence you are bringing to the workshop. When you are in the room, consider if you are present. That may make a difference in your experience."

Although I said "thank you" aloud, in my mind I thought: *I know I was not present. I am barely staying awake in my life and it is taking everything in me to try to focus on each practice. I have no idea how to be present right now because I have no energy.* When we finished speaking, she let me know I could go get my things. It felt like a walk of shame. A few students greeted me with delight. Once they saw me rolling up my mat, the questions started. I gave very vague short answers and tried to leave as quickly as possible. I didn't want to break out in tears again. I made it to my car, but once inside its safety, I burst into sobs. I was so distraught at not being able to finish the workshop. On the way home, I had to pull over to compose myself. I was not good at failing, and I confused it with my self-worth. My entire body ached with an intense feeling of my inadequacies.

I walked through my cousin's door completely defeated. With no plans for the rest of the day, everything felt blank. My canvas had been wiped clean. But I simply did not have the strength to start anything new again. All of this was completely unknown to my cousin's three-year-old son Raylan, who ran up to me at the door and excitedly asked, "Pretzel, swings?!"

I nodded tiredly—he was so excited, there was no way I could say no.

Pretzel was the nickname that he made for me when we were teaching him everyone's names at the kitchen table one day. I went around the table and pointed to each person as he repeated the name. "Mommy," I said aloud as I pointed in the direction of his mother.

"Mommy," he repeated sweetly.

"Daddy."

"Daddy," he repeated clearly.

"Ryan."

"Ryan!" he exclaimed and always made it seem like he was the favorite, which I couldn't help but laugh at.

"Sarah," I said pointing to myself.

"Pretzel," he replied matter of factly.

"Sarah," I repeated.

"Pretzel," he said again. And the name just stuck.

As he swung, his sweet laughter began to ease the despair in my heart. Over my first year in Houston, he had brightened many of my days. You couldn't be sad when you heard his genuine full-body laugh. It was infectious. As I relaxed into the moment, I took notice of the picture-perfect morning and felt comforted by the breeze that blew gently as the sun warmed my skin. I was struck with the realization that the morning might still be wonderful, after all. I could still feel the stinging humiliation of failure, but this moment, well, it was heaven on earth. As I pumped my legs and let myself fly, I committed to taking the workshop next year if I was still in Houston. I would try again. It was going to be possible to heal.

"Pretzel, I want to spell!" I smiled and thought about a word that he could learn to spell that would also capture this moment.

"Love," I offered. We weren't leaving heaven anytime soon.

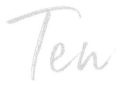

Then

I was living in a world of seemingly polar opposites. My days and nights were split between the environments of one of the world's largest, structured corporations, and a small, organic entrepreneurial yoga studio. At ExxonMobil the culture was competitive. You were expected to be self-sufficient. The company controlled your career moves and there would be little notice when you were about to be promoted. You would learn that you were being placed in a role you knew nothing about, and you had two weeks at most to get your footing. I cannot even count how many times I heard coworkers say it's a "sink or swim" culture. Luckily, adapting quickly is one of my greatest strengths; one of which was noticed by the company and always listed as a positive on my performance reports. This culture only improved my resilience. But it was not without stress!

At the end of each year every employee was ranked from top to bottom. I was always ranked right at the edge of the top category. Throughout the year I would achieve great accomplishments and still be given feedback on seemingly minute details. The expectation was perfection. All details were constantly being scrutinized. *Did you notice the blue in your PowerPoint graph didn't show up as dark when projected? Next time, practice projecting in the conference room before the meeting and check your colors.* It seemed like no matter what I accomplished, it was never enough. *Great job getting that done. Next time be more assertive. There is an impression that you are always just kind.* There was always a feeling that you could not succeed. *Didn't you notice the plant manager wanted to leave early? You need to read the room and shorten your presentation if you see a manager is short on time.* I was left feeling just adequate, not stellar. When I drove home, I felt like I was going to live my second life. The one no one in the office knew about. I would walk into the colorful school of Rasa Yoga, inhale the fragrance of peace from the incense, and be reminded that I am way beyond adequate, perhaps even incredible. There was full acceptance for everyone who came through the doors. This is where I learned what being nonjudgmental really looks like. A student could have a complete meltdown in the corner and it was not seen as a reflection of them. They were not forever imprinted with the story of how they broke down. It was recognized that it was a reaction that they had—not who they are. The studio was run by a community, and the leaders had great depth of patience. They would continue to support you even if it was the twentieth time they were explaining the same lesson. Rasa Yoga held a space of acceptance that made me feel confident to go outside my comfort zone. I saw myself start to open up with the nurturing environment. Before long, I had ditched my wardrobe of all black yoga pants. I was now comfortable wearing vibrantly colored pants in all different prints. My favorite became a peacock-patterned pair. This is honestly why I stayed in Houston as long as I did. I could have interviewed and gotten a new job in Los Angeles, but if I had, I may have given up my chance to learn how to choose happiness. Rasa Yoga showed me a new paradigm I had not witnessed before. It was possible to not judge myself and those around me and thrive in any situation. I knew I needed more time to train with them if I wanted to be able to cultivate this inner stillness myself.

When I *think* back on this time, I wonder, *Why didn't I quit my job? Why did I stay in a place that was so far from my ideal life?* With Rasa Yoga, I was starting to see what could be. It's when I *feel* back to this time that I remember. My job was way easier than college, and despite all the pressure, it felt like a vacation compared to being in school. Plus I was getting paid! Comparing a present moment to an insane past can be dangerous. I didn't have any other reality for comparison. I was right out of school in my first job and as far as I knew, this was what professional life looked and felt like. All my coworkers and friends around me were doing the same thing. My friends who went to medical school made my schedule look wide open. We were all working ourselves to death (the irony of this for how we train doctors in medical school is not lost on me). I kept reasoning that the first year will of course be the hardest. I just had to get through my first and *then* things would get better I told myself. Especially after I learned how to live on my own and I wasn't wedding planning, *then* things would be easier. Thinking about *then* can also be dangerous. Once this happens, *then I will be* is not a helpful approach. I recall driving home one night and the radio DJ was discussing a survey that looked at what keeps people from being happy in their jobs. A key finding was people being really great at something they don't enjoy. That resonated with me. Big time. I kept hearing his words and reflecting on whether I didn't enjoy engineering or was it just this role that I didn't enjoy. I added this to my collection of thoughts on life after college.

These were my conscious thoughts. There was also a deeper driving force I was not yet aware enough to see. I was a trained people pleaser and quitting was not going to please anybody. I had learned well that when I succeeded I got more love and approval, and I wanted that love.

I didn't want any more criticism, there was an abundance of that in my life. If I could just succeed, all would be well. This mindset helped me in many situations of life but my biggest strength could also become my biggest weakness when I did not know when to walk away. Rasa Yoga was the first place I would be praised for failing because that meant I was learning. This felt very uncomfortable for me, so in the meantime, I would stick to succeed or die trying.

I looked up after a knock on my office door to see the plant manager quickly pop her head in the door long enough to say, "Hey Sarah, fantastic job presenting today!"

So many mixed messages. I could do this. I only had to make it through the end of the year, *then* I would get a new job and be with Ryan.

Eleven

Year of Me

I was ecstatic to be going on a new adventure as I rolled my little pink luggage, which had been around the world with me, out to my car. After six months of classes at Rasa Yoga, I had signed up for my first yoga retreat—something I had desired to join for a long time! I wanted to experience the joy and camaraderie that I was certain must be felt at a retreat and I knew it would help me to dive deeper into my yoga practice. This weekend healing immersion was just three days long, but it was my first retreat! Auspiciously held at Padma Shakti's house, the owner of Rasa Yoga, and who would eventually become my yoga guru; my teacher and guide in yoga.

Strolling into the entrance of Padma's house, I was in awe at the shiny marble white floors and grand arches between rooms as I stood in the middle of the foyer feeling uncertain of what to expect. Standing in the same place at the end of the retreat, I felt an all encompassing ease from the nurturing escape I needed after so much change in my life. My feet were grounded on the marble and in no rush to return to my complex emotions that awaited me at home. My eyes scanned the whole room watching the other participants eagerly sign up for the next retreat and file out one by one. It seemed to be the thing to do, but I was craving something more transformative than three more days away, and there were words echoing in my head from a yogini in Louisiana who I had practiced next to once during a summer in college. With brown wavy hair, average body build, and a perfect blue matching yoga set that even included the sports bra, she had watched me practice and must have sensed my passion. Before class, in a minimally decorated room with a single plant and buddha sculpture—as if the minimalism was to make room for the vast number of students around us—she turned with frantic energy to her friend, pointed at me, and exclaimed, "Oh! She's one of the Ashtanga yogis that can do all those back-bendy pretzel poses! You won't believe what she can do!" I felt my energy contract some at the space of my heart as I thought about needing to live up to this expectation and not wanting to perform while I practiced. Then she spoke to me directly. Like a switch had flipped, her frantic energy was gone and replaced with steady eye contact. "Have you considered taking the teacher training program here? You have a strong practice; I see you here every day . . . you should think about it." I had not considered this and didn't envision myself in that training. I was so new to yoga that I could only see myself as a student. I wondered why she saw me that way. With an attempt at a humble reply, I politely told her I didn't feel it was for me. "Well, you should take the training for your own personal development even if you don't care to teach. You'll learn a lot about yoga philosophy." Hmmm, now she had my interest! With these words she nearly put her hands on the steering wheel of my life and pointed it in another direction. I had until this point only heard teacher training and now I was hearing yoga history, philosophy, and self-improvement training. This was a game changer. The idea of signing up for training felt familiar to me as I had studied and participated in after-school activities my whole life. To choose to do this to deepen my own self-awareness just for myself with no grades or competition, felt freeing.

She, a lady I crossed paths with briefly and whose name I never knew, planted a hearty seed in my impressionable twenty-year-old mind. I took a mental note and decided that two years after I graduated college, I would seek out a teacher training program. Well, those words had echoed ever since and my mind had been vacillating around the decision to sign up for Rasa Yoga's teacher training. I had always imagined it a few years out of college, which was an arbitrary amount of time I had decided upon with little basis other than speculating that it would take two or three years to be established in my career and ready for training. It is funny how easy it is to create a plan around what we suspect may be needed and then forget in the moment that there is no reason to stick to that if you now know you don't need that extra time and your career will go on just fine. I luckily had overcome this self-imposed timeline understanding that just a few months out of college worked just as well but I was also debating if I could complete the program in a year if I moved to Los Angeles. Especially since there was an eleven-day intensive required to graduate. Although that sounded like a dream to me, I could not imagine using eleven of my fourteen vacation days while in a long-distance relationship for yoga training. Despite so many logistical questions, I kept returning to the fact that I would be foolish not to take this high-quality training in such an advanced community of yogis and yoginis while I had the chance. In a moment of clarity when I felt frozen in time in the dreamy foyer, I dropped all the what-ifs and decided I would find a way. This was the time to take the step toward the goal that had been ringing in my ears for years.

Padma knew by now that I had been pondering this decision for a few months. She knew I was questioning whether this would work with my desire to move in a year. When I handed her my credit card to enroll, she casually stated, "What a wonderful decision for yourself. I know that your life is not exactly as you would want it right now, but why don't you make the most of this year. This can be the year of Sarah."

Bells went off inside me as she swiped my card and waited for it to process. "Yes," I thought, "this will be the year of me!" As I packed up my mat and headed out to my car, the new words echoing in my ears were Padma's words, like a mantra: the year of Sarah . . . the year of Sarah . . . the year of Sarah. Now I had a direction to head in, a purpose, and my training would be the starting point.

As I headed out the door, she left me with one more lesson. "Remember that with every expansion there is a contraction. This is a law of life. When you go home tonight, it may be normal if you feel a little contraction after making such an expansive decision."

In a small, yet pivotal moment that evening, as I retrieved my mail and noticed the envelope containing my new credit card, a realization dawned on me. The cost of the yoga teacher training was beyond my old credit card limit. Until then, the notion of considering my credit limit hadn't crossed my mind, as I had the necessary funds. Alongside selecting a wedding-dress seamstress and our first dance song, I was learning the many lessons of credit card limits, 401(k) strategies, and health insurance options. I'm not sure if I was shaping adulthood or if adulthood was shaping me. Everything was new to me and I didn't know to open a credit card in college to accumulate credit history, so despite having a good salary, my credit limit was near nonexistent. An initial wave of panic tightened my chest and spiked my body. I paused to feel my feet on the floor and took a breath before jumping to conclusions. Stepping back, I saw that the answer this time was in the envelope I was holding. Swiftly, I called Rasa Yoga, asked for the charge to be canceled and added to the new card. This time I was able to recover back to an expanded state pretty quickly, this incident marked the commencement of what I had claimed to be the "Year of Sarah."

As my mind reeled with all the information I was going to learn, I felt a newfound sense of purpose for the upcoming year. Envisioning a transformed version of myself—confident, radiant, and at peace—I unknowingly committed to looking honestly at and acknowledging my inner pain so that I could heal it. I would learn that one has to feel and study their darkness in order to bring forth the light.

This journey would entail larger contractions that would come with this decision to grow to new levels that I couldn't fathom when I handed over my credit card.

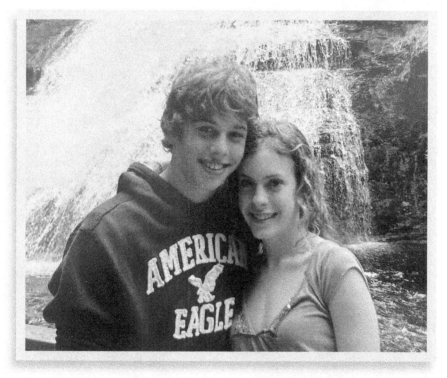

Our first picture together, and we have taken SO many pictures in front of waterfalls since! We were fifteen years old.

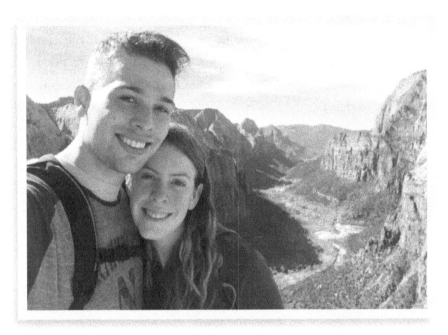

At the top of Angels Landing with Emerald Falls in the background where we got engaged.

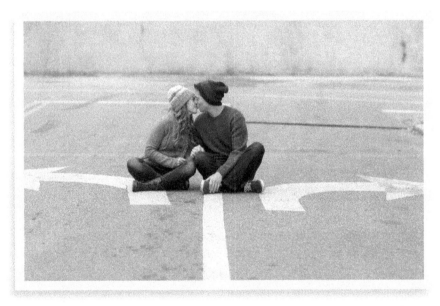

An engagement photo that has always been symbolic of where we were in our lives at that time.

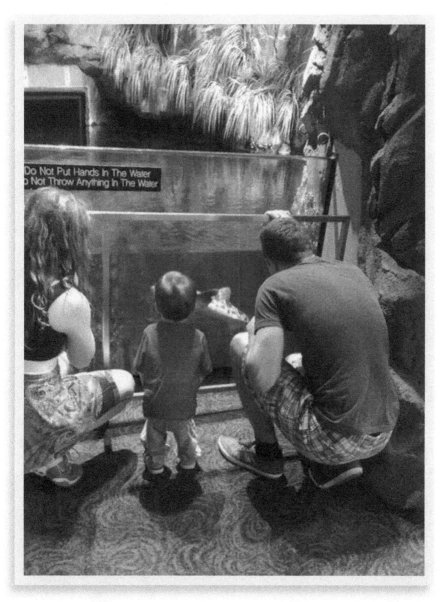

Ryan and me with my cousin Raylan at Moody Gardens Aquarium, watching the seals. Raylan kept excitedly saying, "The puppies are swimming!"

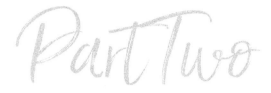

Pain

You have to keep breaking your heart until it opens.

—RUMI

I closed my bedroom door and dropped my bag onto the ground. I was so exhausted. My stomach growled so loudly, it almost echoed against the walls of the empty room—suddenly, I realized I had barely eaten all day and was famished. It was close to midnight, but I pulled a granola bar out of my bag and ate it anyway. As the dry bits of oat stuck in the back of my throat I decided it was probably better than not eating anything. I had been by Ryan's hospital bedside since 7:00 a.m., and my mind kept flashing back to images of him in pain. It was our junior year of high school, and he had been very ill all year. We had been in and out of hospitals constantly, and doctors could not determine a diagnosis. On this day in particular, he had been in excruciating pain, and it had taken over eight hours to even get a doctor to his bedside. It had been so difficult to watch and I felt absolutely helpless. He was in so much pain and the only thing I could do was essentially hold his hand and be there as support. I was not a medical professional, and all my searching online had yielded nothing. I had never questioned being there for him while he was sick. I loved him. I wanted to see him be well again. I wanted to see the radiant energy that had first won me over, come back and fill him with vitality again. Yet everyone around me seemed to have a different opinion. Throughout the year, people were constantly surprised that I was always at the hospital.

"Why are you still with him when he is so sick and you two cannot even do anything?"

"Love is not supposed to make you come home and cry every night."

"You are ruining your last years of high school."

I knew high schoolers were immature, so I took many of their comments with a grain of salt. After all, Ryan did not ask to be sick. He did not try to make our year like this. It was the comments of some adults close to me that really made me question if I was the crazy one. If I was the only one not questioning our relationship, then maybe I was not thinking clearly. Slugging down a glass of water, I headed blindly to my bed. I threw the sheets back and climbed in. I needed a sanity check, desperately. As I drifted off into an exhausted sleep, I was jolted awake when a friend's mom came to mind. She was a psychologist and I could use some wisdom. I held up my phone to check the time. It was well past midnight. Was it too late to call her? Would she be okay with me asking for advice? I flipped open my phone (yes, it was flip phones then) and dialed. My heart pounded as I considered that maybe I was crossing the line, . . . ring . . . ring . . . on the third ring, I was amazed to hear her answer. "Hi, Sarah, how are you?" Her calm voice didn't skip a beat.

"I am sorry to call so late." I gulped as my heart continued to race. "It is just that I was hoping to ask for some advice. Everyone keeps telling me I shouldn't stay with Ryan and that a relationship shouldn't look this sad and tiring. The comments are so frequent that I am starting to question myself . . . I'm wondering . . . am I missing something?"

She kindly replied confidently with a soft, empathetic voice, "Well, I can tell you what I teach my clients. In a relationship, you want to imagine a triangle. It is divided into three parts: Me, We, and They. You always want these parts to be in balance. You need to take care of yourself, you will need to take care of Ryan, and Ryan will need to take care of you. There will be times where one of these will need to be more than the other, but they balance out over time. The question you need to ask yourself is, when Ryan is healthy and capable, does he or will he take care of me?"

"Yes, yes he does and will," I answered without even a shred of hesitation. "Even this year, when he has a good day, he has really made sure to ask how I am doing. He has done everything he can to give back to me." We chatted some more about Ryan's health, and how tired I was, but ultimately, I found so much relief in our conversation. As I hung up the phone, I exhaled all the stress out of my body. I didn't know what was wrong with Ryan, but I did know that our relationship was here to stay. No one could say a word to make me doubt that, from now on.

Twelve

Heartburn

The room was filled with excitement and high-pitched laughter. Twas the night before my bridal shower, and I was sharing a hotel room with Lorena and one of my bridesmaids, Brittney. They both came to every wedding event I had, and their support meant everything to me. Brittney, ever the loyalist, actually drove two hours to the middle-of-nowhere Illinois to pick up my wedding dress at the boutique after I moved to Houston. She later met me, with dress in hand, when I was in Chicago for a business trip. It had taken nine months for my dream dress to arrive so I was not about to risk it being lost in checked luggage—it was too precious, so I had decided to carry it back with me on the plane and make sure it never left my side. I chuckled to myself again, as I pictured two of our groomsmen helping me shove my beautiful wedding gown with ten layers of tulle into my tiny carry-on luggage. As I stood in line for security, I prayed that I would not get a random luggage check at the airport, because I was pretty certain I wouldn't be able to get my dress back into the luggage alone. It was a relief when I was finally back in Houston and I could gaze at my dress, safely hung up in my room.

As our conversation drifted into sleep, I tossed and turned as I became increasingly uncomfortable with the worst heartburn I had ever experienced. I had only ever had it a few times in my life and never this extreme. As I struggled to find a comfortable position to sleep in it felt like a hole was going to burn right through my throat as I lay in the hotel bed. I scanned the room and could see Lorena and Brittney were both sound asleep, so I grabbed the room key and snuck out of the room as quietly as I could, hoping I would not wake them. On the hunt for a vending machine, I was so happy to spot Tums in the hotel lobby. I quickly pressed the buttons on the machine to deliver a pack, and as I approached our room, I was shocked to realize I had eaten the whole sleeve of antacid. Despite overdosing on calcium, I found little to no relief. If an entire sleeve of Tums had not even dented the symptoms, I knew I just had to surrender to the night. I'd go back upstairs and try to fall asleep. If nothing else, I could rest a little. As the hole continued to burn into the flesh of my throat, questions flooded my mind all night to figure out the cause. My cousin, and matron of honor, had to stay at home because she was sick. Had I picked up what she had? Or was it something I ate? I reviewed everything I had eaten that day to no avail. What had I done that would cause this inferno?

I barely slept that night and was feeling pretty rough the next morning. It was fortuitous that a wedding makeup trial was planned before the shower to heavily cover up any bags under my eyes with foundation. I pretended to be awake while greeting all the family who had come to celebrate. About an hour in, I found a moment of rest, a break from catching everyone up on my life, and sat down to enjoy some cake. My fork pierced the slice of confection as I anticipated taking the next sweet bite right when I got a text from my work backfill. It was terrible luck, but my role had a lot of important tasks taking place on this particular weekend and I was forced to leave everything under a coworker's watchful eye. In the midst of hosting fifty guests, I shot back a text with how to reach the furnace expert who would have all the answers they needed and then went back to faking being awake while I opened presents. I felt a responsibility to hide how terrible I was feeling; everyone had put in so much effort to be there, for me. But the faking was literally taking everything out of me.

When I landed in Houston Sunday night, I was unbelievably exhausted. All I could do was sleep. On Monday, I learned there was a close safety incident on the startup of the furnace I had received the text about. The overall consensus was that I had not provided enough guidance to my coworker who had supported me. My operations lead pulled me into his office, he was irate. "Sarah, that furnace startup could have ended really badly this weekend. If we had not shut it down, that kind of error could injure or kill people. It is my job to make sure these things never happen. What happened?"

I didn't know the right words to say. I knew this was a sensitive situation and I obviously regretted what had happened. I took a deep breath and spoke from my heart. "I know. I am really sorry. It would never be my intention to hurt someone," I said sincerely but quietly. I felt a softening from him—almost a sigh.

"Yeah, I know you never intended that, Sarah. Let's be careful going forward." I walked away feeling nervous. I couldn't tell if he really forgave me, and I knew my work was going to be scrutinized more than the already intense level going forward. My heartburn was still very much there. It no longer seemed to be from something I ate, and my energy was being further drained.

Over the next few weeks I learned that there are a lot of options when it comes to over-the-counter heartburn medications. I experimented with some and while I sometimes thought they were helping, they really weren't effective. My throat felt like a raging forest fire all the time, and I only had Dixie cups of water to put it out.

I don't remember when the burping started, but slowly, out of nowhere, I developed a constant burp. It was not a belch, but a very consistent burp that never went away. It was like an internal water torture system, and I felt like I was nearing the edge of sanity with each burp. It was typically hard to fall asleep, and when I did, I would wake up in the middle of the night with intense pain under my heart in the middle of my rib cage from an air bubble. Pressure would build up and I would have to burp to get rid of the pain in order to fall back asleep. After weeks of this torture, I sought out a gastroenterologist as my symptoms seemed to only be getting worse; I was desperate to feel better. The doctor conducted a thorough examination and sent me off for an endoscopy. I was so eager to get my results; anything to feel better! I sat on the edge of the medical room chair in anticipation of the mystery reveal only to be informed that they had found nothing. As it turned out, the doctor didn't know what was causing my symptoms anymore than I did. Everything looked perfect, the blood work even came back normal, and he was out of ideas. I was deeply disappointed. My hope dimmed as he sent me home with some stronger heartburn medicine and essentially wished me good luck.

Out of desperation, I started my own research on the internet. Never a great idea. There were all sorts of suggestions, especially around testing for food allergies. Many things I read suggested elimination diets; a week of no dairy followed up by a week with no gluten, and so on, to see if it was a specific food group that was causing my misery. I decided to try some of these, but none panned out. What I did notice was that the burping got worse after I ate literally anything. Slowly, I started skipping dinner until I no longer ate after 2:00 p.m. This was the only way I found I could sleep instead of staying up burping all night. Because of my empty stomach, the mornings were an oasis of peace and as I watched the clock, I would dread having to eat breakfast. I had quickly gone from living to eat to eating to live.

Over the next few months, I went to several doctors and continued to leave without answers. I remember going to a homeopath, a holistic healthcare practitioner, and telling him my story. He looked up from his notes and asked, "Have you lost any weight because of this?" When I told him I had lost eight pounds already, he replied, "This is very serious. That is a lot." His matter of fact tone was empathetic as he stood up and went to his back room. He returned with a vial of three very tiny white dots covered in solution which I would much later learn are sugar balls to hold the homeopathic medicine he prescribed for me. He explained that I was to take these, and my burping should stop. It did stop, for half a day. But that was it. Between paying out of pocket and not knowing what was actually in the medicine, I decided not to return. I sometimes wonder if I might have found relief sooner if I had been willing to pay out of pocket.

One day I came across an article on the bacteria *Helicobacter pylori* or H. pylori for short. The titles of all the websites on it had the words *excessive burping*. My heart raced as I read through the website; it perfectly described my symptoms. I really believed this was my answer, and was frustrated when all my doctors dismissed my claim. I was told that H. pylori was very rare; there was little chance that what I had was this condition. I was desperate and not ready to put this aside so easily. I'd been sick for months and this was the closest thing I had come to an answer. I kept asking around about it, and learned that I could get tested without a doctor's script. With so much hope in my heart, I burped all the way to the testing site and was flabbergasted when the results said I was negative for the H. pylori bacteria. Although I knew it was a good thing not to have this bacteria, I was in disbelief, really, denial. If it was not that, then what did I have? I went back to my online research, and discovered it was common to have a false negative. I still slightly clung to my theory that I might have this bacteria and the treatment for it would end my misery. I needed a glimmer of hope that I could eventually return to full health. It would happen, but I had to manage in this condition for many more months first.

The main issue I faced was constant fatigue. I was having trouble falling asleep, but more than that, my digestion was poor. Ayurveda, the sister science to yoga, says that the health of our digestion is directly related to our overall health. Stomachs can be likened to the engine of a car. Trying to thrive everyday with poor digestion was like trying to race a car with an engine held together with bubblegum and rubber bands. My days weren't pretty or efficient, but I kept going. I still had big plans I was passionate about and I wasn't about to stop.

I do wish I had slowed down enough to realize the word *heart* is part of heartburn.

Thirteen

Not Equal

I listened in a half daze, detached from the conversation in the room. My body was sitting in the same chair, at the long table which our entire team sat at every morning for the operations meeting, but mentally, I wasn't there. It was like some safety feature had kicked in so I couldn't be hurt further. The words just went through me. "What? We're not going to be able to do that. I need at least four weeks' lead time to be able to order the material. You never told me this was needed until now." I couldn't believe what I was partly hearing, and sadly I could at the same time. The worst part was the operations lead was looking at me with direct eye contact as he spoke. For a long time, ever since I kept my car instead of trading it in for a truck, I had suspected that I was being framed to look like I was not doing my work. The manipulation was sometimes so subtle that I also felt I was being paranoid or overthinking. But yesterday cleared up everything.

I had gone to his office to discuss the upcoming maintenance items and we had reviewed all the logistics. The details were input into the computer and we were squared away. We kept talking about random other topics and something led me to say, "Oh no, I have faith."

"Now, that is not a word I have heard in a while," he answered immediately. The tone took me by surprise and I knew I had accidentally entered dangerous territory. I had meant that I trusted everything would work out but I could tell that it had been interpreted to imply religion. My intention didn't matter and he asked about my beliefs around God. This was not a good conversation to get into at work so I skirted the question and tried to divert to another topic. My attempt at diverting to another topic was met with another diversion. "You probably also believe men and women are equal too, huh," his statement was disguised as a question. "Well, yes I do believe men and women should be treated equally," I replied since I did strongly believe this.

"But they are not equal. They are physically different and that cannot be argued."

"What does that mean to you? That they should be treated differently?" I asked.

"It means men and women were built to do different things so their roles are different," he replied without hesitation. I was pretty stunned at his direct language. It was at this point that I had my answer: I was not wanted in this job because he believed that it really should be done by a man. Overwhelmed by the ick factor, my nerves got the best of me, and I cut the exchange short by making up some sort of excuse as to why I needed to get back to my office. I left the building as quickly as I could, drove to my office, and ignored the open door policy as I shut my door to be alone. All I could think about was how it was not in my head; I really was not being welcomed.

I was not sure what to do next and it took me some time to get grounded in my decision. A few days passed and then I got up the courage to tell a superior what had been said to me and that I felt I was being mistreated. They dismissed me with full disbelief. Their response included stories of how well they knew his sweet family.

He treats his family, especially his daughters, so well!

The sentence must have just been taken out of context because there is no way he would have intended it that way.

Sarah, get to know him better as a person.

I had no doubt that he is an endearing dad and husband, but I was not family.

I would continue to reflect on what to do next.

But now I knew. I knew I was not paranoid and I knew why my body felt so heavy each morning as I got up to drive to my morning meeting. I drowned even further in regret that I had not followed my heart on what job to accept out of college.

Fourteen

Falling Foolishly

One day I was sitting in the office of one of the supervisors in my hall. We had developed a good relationship and I respected her. She had called me in to ask if she could offer some feedback. In my usual fashion, I welcomed all feedback even if I knew it might be hard to hear. She gently prefaced her feedback with how it is her job to observe the young engineers and see how they are performing as well as interacting with the team. With me, she had noticed that I really connected and established a relationship with the engineers in the hall, but there was more I could do to establish a stronger rapport with operations. This was followed up with a suggestion to come to work earlier because the operations team really respects when people come in early to chat ahead of the meeting even if it doesn't seem to directly help my job.

I knew she was right. I had been aware of this for a while. There were just a few issues and hesitations on my end. The toxic culture I was confronting and my health. As politely as I could, I agreed with her and instead of responding with a politically correct answer, I explained how I was having trouble getting in earlier with my stomach issues. That was not what I wanted to say, but it was an honest answer. I waited in nervous anticipation of her response. I had never spoken this honestly at work.

As a friend, I saw empathy in her eyes. As a supervisor, I saw concern in her eyes. I felt very vulnerable. I wanted to respond with a resounding yes and add reassurance that I would immediately start coming in earlier. But that just was not going to happen. My emotional shell had cracked enough that some authenticity shined through. Perhaps it was the trust I had in our relationship. Perhaps it was desperation. Perhaps it was a baby step to becoming wise. Many would say it was foolish.

Whether it was a moment of wisdom is up for debate, but I do know I was learning through experience that perfectionism does not work. It is not real.

Later that month, my worst work fear finally came to be. I had been up all night burping and could not fathom how I would go to work. I called my supervisor at 6:00 a.m. to let her know my situation. At least up to this point, I had never missed work. I had been struggling, but I had upheld all my responsibilities, so this was an unsettling phone call for me. I did not want to have to ask for time off or be seen in a less than optimal light. Now, I had made the call I never wanted to. She told me to take the day to rest and that I could silence my phone. The team would cover for me. I just needed to let her know how I was at the end of the day. It was not my ideal scenario—in fact anything but that—but I had the day off. I learned I actually really needed the rest. It ended up being one of the best calls I made for myself that year and it was not as fatal as I had imagined it would be. I had only taken one day off the entire year because I needed to save vacation days for our wedding and honeymoon. I needed a break on many levels. I put aside all work and wedding planning that day. To not be on call, even for a day, was a blessing. I felt like a weight had been lifted off my shoulders. I was practically floating. I went to a natural food store that day to see if they had anything that may help my predicament. As I opened the door to leave, I felt a spacious freedom as the sun was shining down on me. I felt happiness from feeling the sun's rays on my skin and taking a deeper breath than I had in a long time. I hadn't even realized how hard it had gotten to breathe with the weight I was carrying. Looking back, it seems I should have been able to understand more of what was going on with my health from my reaction that day, but sometimes lessons have to play themselves out until we can see clearly.

The next morning I picked back up the weight and reluctantly turned on my phone.

Fifteen

Learning to Fail

One night I found myself sitting on the tiled floor of Ryan's bathroom and not only could I not stop burping but it was getting worse with each passing hour. I couldn't fall asleep so I went to the bathroom to not wake him up. It was Saturday night and looking back, I am sure that is what escalated all of my symptoms. I had a hyper case and slightly nuanced version of the Sunday scaries. Every ounce of my being did not want to fly home the next day. I wanted to stay in California and laugh with Ryan every night about our day's adventures. As I sat there I began to cry because I had no more strength. It was such a low feeling as I observed how I had lost my health and normalcy. After a bit, Ryan walked into the bathroom asking what was wrong. I just kept sobbing and saying how tired I was and that I could not fall asleep. I had reached complete exhaustion and felt pathetic. He hugged me empathetically in a way that also said something has got to change. We both knew that but we didn't know how. The next day I inevitably had to catch my flight and I recall wishing so much I had the energy to read on the flight as I love that uninterrupted time to indulge myself. Even then I was trying to optimize my time, but all I could do was rest.

I feel embarrassed when I reflect on where I was during this year. It can be difficult to admit. I never dreamed I would have a breakdown over our separation. I think I felt that nothing big enough had happened for me to feel this low. It's easy to judge myself for not making changes faster, but I know the emotion came from so much more than our long distance. I was learning how to transition from college to work, live in a new state, plan a wedding, be apart from the love of my life, complete a yoga training, field others' judgments, and most importantly, find my voice. There was a slow and long build up of many factors that all crashed into each other. I didn't have enough life experience to know or courage to learn that if I stood up for what I needed or took a few weeks off work to rest, that everything would be perfectly okay. Is this what people mean when they say adulting is hard? I sometimes wish I could rewrite it and paint myself differently. If only that could change or help anything. This denial would only make it worse. I know the best thing I can do for myself is to see my past self in her entirety. To be willing to see my full history honestly. Look my younger self right in the eyes and say, "I love you. I know you are doing your best. I wish you could see the larger picture already. You will get through this. Thank you for doing the hard work. I see you. I see you fully. I will not look away. I forgive you."

When I reflect honestly, I was angry, sad, lonely, confused, resentful, attached, hopeful. I was heartbroken by the wild story playing in my head. I was allowing myself to think that I was left behind in Texas while Ryan got to live my California dream. This was of course false because Ryan didn't even want to live in California. It wasn't his dream, and I imagine he would have preferred to be staying with family members in the suburbs like me. I had anger that I didn't know how to process. I was hanging on like people in movies who have just fallen off a cliff and somehow grabbed hold of a lone tree limb by their fingertips. They are fierce and put their entire focus into hanging on with the belief that they can somehow lift their bodyweight back up to safety. I was not able to pull myself back up the ledge. I held on for a long time, because I feared failure. Luckily, I eventually fell and then learned to walk back to the top. Padma reminded me that it is through failure that we learn. We rise up from our lowest lows. If we are not failing then we are not pushing our boundaries. It was through my yoga training that I came to appreciate this failure. I slowly came to realize that failure is a part of success. You cannot have one and not the other. A lack of failure indicates that the goals being set are not challenging enough. Success requires walking into the unknown and outside of our comfort zone. That is what makes the victory so sweet because you have actually made it through something difficult. Who has ever felt triumphant completing something easy?

I forgive me.

I forgive me.

I forgive me.

Sixteen

Wedding Day

Our wedding week arrived. Throughout the year, I had really hoped that I would not be sick by the time of our wedding. In my mind, I was always going to be healed before then, but life unfolded differently from my imagination. I still had heartburn. I still had burping. In fact, I had lost so much weight that my wedding dress was slightly baggy. When the fittings were originally completed, it was so tight that I could barely sit down. Well, I could not sit down, it was truly form fitted—we ended up buying a second dress so I could sit during the reception—but by the time the wedding rolled around I was swimming in my dress. I clearly recall that I spent time the night before flying to our wedding mentally preparing myself that nothing could stop my wedding day from being the best day ever. By this time, I had gone from being in retreats to full blown yoga training and I had been learning how my thoughts and vocabulary shape my entire experience. One of the largest realizations I had embodied was that we do not see the world as it really is, we see the world through our perspective. Two people can live the same day and yet undergo entirely contrasting experiences based on their mindsets. One shift I had been working with to become more expansive was replacing the words *I have to* with *I get to*. I found this small shift made a radical change in my inspiration levels and how I felt. It's the difference between *I have to pay my apartment rent* and *I get to pay my apartment rent to live in a safe and cozy place* or *I have to go to the grocery* and *I get to choose what I would like to eat and not worry about finding food*. The last few weeks leading up to my wedding had been difficult, but I knew that did not have to impact the wedding. I was determined to enjoy life. I applied my yoga training even further and eliminated the words *I have to* from my thoughts. I wrote in my journal:

I GET TO go to my wedding during a difficult time!

I GET TO connect with my family and friends!

I GET TO live in Houston!

I GET TO overcome obstacles everyday!

My happiness did not depend on a healthy stomach and I was gracious that I would *get to* do so many important things in one day with people I love! I was genuinely eager to finally call Ryan my husband. We had been together eight years and I had learned that people do not take you seriously with the word boyfriend. When I referred to my boyfriend, I could feel people thinking, "Yeah, there will be a new one next month or next year." I tried to convey that we were serious, but it rarely mattered. It didn't help that we were so young either. Somehow, declaring you are married eliminates the judgment that you are young and naive.

We both had to fly to our big day because we chose to get married in Ohio. My papa had lost hearing in one ear and the doctors believed he would lose hearing in both if he flew. I couldn't imagine my wedding day without my papa there, and honestly Ryan could not either as he had been adopted as a grandson with us meeting so young. In some ways, this was my home. I had spent a month each summer in Ohio with my grandparents and as much as my family moved and evolved, we always returned there to see family for the holidays—even Ryan since we had been seventeen. We'd walk into the brick room entrance welcomed by the familiar fireplace and be mesmerized by the snow covered pine trees peeking through the large kitchen window. Grandma and Papa's house may not have been where I lived but it was our extended home, so we planned our wedding near my grandparents' town. This always added a fun layer to people guessing where our wedding was located and inevitably being perplexed that it was not in New Jersey, Illinois, Texas, California, or a destination wedding. When I landed in Ohio our wedding planner said she had the same stomach issue as me and I *must* go to her holistic medicine practitioner. Hearing that someone had the same symptoms brought another spark of hope for me and it was probably pretty easy for me to get inspired before my wedding. We booked an appointment the morning before our dress rehearsal, and my mom and Ryan came with me as this holistic healer hooked wires up to me and all sorts of bars and squiggles appeared on a screen. With all three of us being engineers, we were looking intently trying to figure out how this probe with wires was outputting these numbers and what in the world the graph was saying? Our analyzing brains were trying so hard when the healer announced she had my diagnosis. I held my breath as she explained that I had several strains of bacteria living in my stomach, including E. coli. I immediately started to think about raw chicken and rotten spinach, which made me physically flinch with anxiety, but I brought myself back to regulation when I remembered I had been living with this for a long time without violently vomiting. "Shouldn't I be violently ill?" I asked. She explained that lower amounts of bacteria don't always react in that way. She recommended natural herbs that I needed to take in order to clear all of this up. She sent me home with many bottles of tablets and a regimen of what to take before every meal. There were fourteen different horse-sized tablets to ingest before every meal for the next month. When I put them together they didn't even fit in my hand. As I choked them down, I pleaded with the Universe that they would take effect before our wedding the next day.

I GET TO take handfuls of tablets!

I GET TO try something new!

I GET TO bring these on my honeymoon!

I GET TO enjoy the day no matter what else is happening! I reminded myself as I swallowed the last pill.

Our wedding day came, and it was like a fairytale come true. Each aspect of the wedding had meaning for us. The reception began with a college friend singing "Ave Maria" in German. This was arranged to honor the fact that my mom had also had a college friend sing "Ave Maria" at her wedding and that Ryan and I had met in German class. While wedding planning, Mom and I agreed we wanted the guests to have a memorable experience from their first step into the venue; we wanted them to be mesmerized from the moment they walked through the door. We hoped their first impression would be in awe of the beauty all around them. The plan was to have two swan ice sculptures on either side of the staircase leading up to the table with the guest book placed next to a large flower display. The ice sculptures were a requirement because I had grown up hearing my grandma continually say how she regretted not having ice sculptures at my mom's wedding. We were able to heal a thirty-year-old family wound for her by having them at my wedding. I think she is now at peace with having missed them at my mom's. The sculptures and flowers would have been more than enough, but in passing, I mentioned a cherished childhood memory to my mom that I had of going to the Biltmore Estate in middle school as part of a family vacation. We had visited during the holidays and when we opened the doors to the mansion, I was enveloped by warmth and my attention was captivated by the stunning sight of four majestic gold harps sitting in the center of the grand, high-ceiling atrium. The women gracefully strummed the harps filling the expansive space with their melodious music. It was unforgettable and so, of course, my mom remembered when I mentioned it. She responded by saying she could look into this to see if we could get four harps. I hadn't meant that we needed to recreate this—it was just the strongest memory I had for creating an epic entrance, but now that I had resurfaced this moment, my mom graciously decided we would try to recreate this for our guests.

My mom really poured her heart into our wedding. She took care of the majority of the logistics and helped with everything. She even found four harpists to play at the entrance as guests arrived, and in a place like Dayton, Ohio, it was no easy feat. She was like a magician pulling that stunt off, and I was grateful as it set an amazing tone for the wedding.

The best things in life you cannot plan. During the ceremony, Ryan started crying as "Here Comes the Bride" played while I walked down the aisle. He continued to cry throughout the entire ceremony. Given that he was the only person miked, everyone knew. It was without a doubt the best part of our entire wedding. I knew how deep his love ran, and on our wedding day, he put it proudly on display to all our family and friends. He showed his depth of love for me with his vulnerability as it seemed like all his feelings could no longer be kept inside. I do believe being long distance all year added to this buildup. His emotion surprised and moved everyone in the room.

We actually have Ryan on video a year before our wedding saying that he cannot wait to see me sobbing when we read our vows. It turns out, he was the one who sobbed and I was so happy that I could not stop smiling. There was just one moment during my vows that I choked up. I promised, "I will never let you wake up alone because you will always be in my mind and in my heart." This struck a chord deep in my soul. This sentence could be read as a cliché line, but for us, there was endless meaning packed into those words. We had learned over that last year that we could promise each other we would always be there, even if we could not physically be there.

Our entire day was a beautiful celebration of coming together. We were both there physically, and our family and friends from all stages of our life were gathered. High school friends from New Jersey, college friends from Northwestern, grad school friends from UCLA, coworkers from ExxonMobil, family friends from Ohio, and extended family from all over America came. It was a true celebration of our life, the path we took to get to that moment, and a pause in time to honor the journey we had yet to live together.

We escaped to an all inclusive resort in Jamaica for a week afterwards, and it was everything you hope for on a honeymoon. We watched other couple's weddings from the hot tub, snorkeled in the afternoons, and read books reclined by the ocean. We let ourselves forget life back at home—more accurately our homes—during this pause. When it was time to resume life, leaving was painful. It was clear by now that every natural herb known to man was not going to heal me, and maybe E. coli was not my issue. I had been taking the handfuls of pills as prescribed and the holistic healer said it should show a pretty immediate effect, but my symptoms were the same as they had been for months. Seeing Ryan had helped me to focus less on my symptoms, and this was the longest we had been together in the last year. It felt joyous. Now I had to go home, and not only was I leaving Ryan, but I was going back to live in a new home. The timing just happened to work out best if I moved out of my cousin's house then and it was an unfortunate series of events. Our flights home both had a connection through North Carolina, which seemed like such a random airport to me. This luckily meant we at least got to leave Jamaica together and buy some more time. As we walked side by side down the terminal after we landed in America, it felt like time had slowed down. It crossed my mind repeatedly that I should just find a seat on Ryan's flight and go to California with him to start our married life. But I'm not the type of person to not show up to work, and as much as I wanted to just go home with him, old habits die hard.

As we walked down the center of the hallway, clutching each other's hands, it felt like we were the only people there. The airport was filled with people going everywhere, but in my mind, they were just flashes of color and energy. My memory of this moment is crystal clear, down to the details of the embroidery of my gray shirt. Everyone was happier than us, and as my eyes scanned the room for another sad couple to connect with, I locked in on a familiar face. Blonde and lean, she was leaning against a railing in a relaxed tree pose, or perhaps she was just resting her right foot on her left shin and I couldn't see past my yoga lens. As I continued to stare, my eyes landed on her mala necklace—which was a telltale sign that she was indeed a yogini.

"Ryan, I know her. Come this way." I pointed in the direction of the blonde in tree pose, but Ryan had already identified her mala and put it together.

It was not lost on me that I was in a moment of pure sadness, and out of nowhere, the Universe had placed one of my favorite yoga teachers right directly in front of me. Even though it was out of character for me to approach a celebrity, I felt like I had some sort of duty to myself and the cosmos to go up and express my gratitude for all she didn't know she had done for me.

"Are you Kino MacGregor?" I asked tentatively when I had gotten within a few feet of her. I hoped I was coming across with a calm demeanor even though I was bursting inside. Kino is an internationally known Ashtanga yogini who is the youngest woman to be certified to teach the lineage from the founder Sri Pattahbi Jois. She had been an inspiration for me along my own yoga journey.

"Yes, I am," she answered with a smile that conveyed she was surprised to be recognized in this smaller airport.

"It is so great to meet you!" I gushed. "I follow you and really appreciate what you have shown is possible for women in yoga. Thank you for sharing it with us." I had one of those moments where I realized I had no plan for what I was going to say. I took note that I need to be ready with what I want to say if I ever meet a role model again.

Kino thanked me for the kind words and asked some about my yoga training. I was still so surprised to run into her. Seeing her made me feel a tiny bit closer to the ancient yoga lineages. It also made a very heavy day, a little lighter. My meeting her could be seen as coincidence or silly but I felt it had meaning, and it is us in the end who give meaning to our experiences. I chose to give meaning to this chance encounter, so therefore it was meaningful, right or wrong. I took it as a sign that I needed to go home to Texas where my guru was and keep practicing yoga. I was being called to dive deeper into this philosophy and trust that there was more there for me on my journey.

This encounter also provided me something else to think about that day instead of what was ahead. I held onto this moment when Ryan and I had to say goodbye, as I landed in Houston, and as I took an Uber back to my new home.

I GET TO go back to Houston and learn from a master yogini, Padma.

Seventeen

Loneliness

It was pretty surreal to move into a new place right after my honeymoon. I arrived around midnight and the house was pitch black. A fellow yogini and consultant who was only home one weekend a month, let me rent her home, and this was not the one weekend she was in town. Since I was not too familiar with the layout or light switches, I placed my hand on the wall and followed the twists and turns in the dark to find my way to my room. Alone in this darkness, I imagined what it must feel like to come home together after the honeymoon and open wedding presents together. I made up that there would be laughter and we would immediately use the pancake griddle when opened no matter what time of day. How different it would be. As I slipped into my new bed, I thanked my past self for dealing with the mattress saga where the wrong mattress was delivered three times and not dismissing it for wedding planning, so I could now sleep soundly. That is certainly a night I will never forget. Everything so new and unfamiliar with the paradox of being alone after a trip to get married amongst all my family and friends. These moments are definitely some of the more challenging times in a long-distance relationship where sadness creeps in. I went to work the next day with very little sleep and while it was an average day for others, I was processing a lot of emotion while completing my tasks. My life had shifted even if it did not look that way externally.

That whole week, I lived out of a suitcase as I moved over my belongings, dreaming of the day I would move my belongings into a house where both Ryan and I would live. That day was not fast enough for the people around me as I found we once again surprised the people in our lives. It turned out that a large majority assumed we would move in together after the big day. It also turned out that we assumed it was obvious that wasn't happening. If we were going to end our long-distance relationship, we wouldn't have waited for a ceremony. We were apart because we were supporting each other's aspirations not because we were waiting for documentation to declare us a legal entity. We were ironically once again disappointing others taking the path less traveled although it felt to us like we were just continuing on the same path.

"When are you moving in together?"

"Have you gotten a new job?"

"Can Ryan finish his degree from Houston?"

"What is your guys' plan?"

"Have you started house searching?"

"Well, you can finally get back together!"

"Which place have you two decided to live in?"

These questions came with an extra harshness this time. People were not as forgiving. You'd think we were doing something blasphemous. I found that long distance has been somewhat accepted for younger couples, especially if one is in the military. Being married *and* long distance on the other hand is far from being accepted culturally. This was another layer of us truly learning to not weigh others' opinions of us into our self-worth or happiness. We had to look inward and remember our choice was valid. It seems we have collectively decided you are only successful if you buy a house with a white picket fence and have at least two children. When did we decide this? Who created this idea? Why do so many of us follow this expectation? Where in this formula is making sure we are happy? What is the toll that this is taking on people who do not find or want this? How long are we going to keep hurting people by judging them against an arbitrary belief?

Do I hope we can start being less critical of how people choose to spend their lives and not benchmark them against an arbitrary ideal? Do I promise to try to be less critical of people in sickness and in health?

I do.

There were nights that I closed my eyes to pretend Ryan was there because, inevitably, it was at night when my loneliness was the greatest. It didn't matter how much we had communicated in the day or how well-crafted my life was, the loneliness always surfaced. And for me, the deeper my love, the more loneliness I felt—true love seemed to have opened a portal to a place where I felt not only its ethereal uplift, but all other emotions intensely as well. The more I have experienced love in my life, the more I have felt the full spectrum of emotions with greater intensity. It is like the reservoir for which I can hold this connected network of "feels" expands with the force of love—a network that includes sadness.

There were many nights when I felt a deep sadness. It felt dark. It felt like there was a deep void I could not fill. A hunger. Often, sadness showed itself late at night when I was at home. In the beginning before I had heartburn, I sometimes confused it for actual hunger and would eat late at night. My favorite food of choice was always oatmeal. It was warm and soft as it filled my stomach with comfort. Over time, I learned to let myself feel the sadness fully. It took time for me to realize I was meant to feel it completely. I slowly grew to where I could remember I feel lonely, but I am not lonely. I feel sad, but I am not sad. They did not define me. I just felt them and I must feel them. I often did not want to feel this energy, but had learned too well that if I didn't, they would manifest themselves eventually anyway, often in a significantly worse way. Emotion is energy in motion and if I stopped the motion, it was going to show up later as muscle tension, burping, or deeper emotion. Numbing it did not work. That only caused an accumulation that led to more suffering. The poet Hāfez says it best, "Don't surrender your loneliness so quickly. Let it cut more deep. Let it ferment and season you as few human or even divine ingredients can."

For me, I found the best way to feel the deep sadness was to allow myself to cry. I would let the tears come and sink fully into loneliness. I personally love the R.E.M song "Everybody Hurts." I would play that song and really feel it. It would resonate with my mood. Honestly the tone and words are so beautiful. It creates such a sorrowful tone with the lovely reminder that if you are human, everybody hurts at some point. You feel lonely but you are not alone. We all face this challenge. We all cry.

As I started allowing myself to feel my sadness, the friendlier we became. I saw that it had something to teach me. One day when I was feeling down because I had just dropped Ryan off at the airport, I wrote in my journal, "There is something beautiful about sadness. I do not know how to describe the sensation, but without deep love and passion it does not exist. And if you can go through it to heal, then beautiful things grow out of the sadness." I believe I was starting to understand that emotions do not actually reveal if something is good or bad; that I've simply been taught to associate what feeling goes with right or wrong through societal constructs. And in this understanding, I was starting to grasp that my loneliness and sadness were neither good nor bad, they *just* were, and these misconceptions were based on judgment and time; they weren't real. I was learning that there is a real sweetness to sadness; the realization that somethings in life are temporary. It seems I was baby-stepping my way with this understanding because realizing that everything is temporary all at once might have been too much for me to bear, so I had to do it one sad episode at a time because truly mastering nonattachment takes practice. In Sanskrit, the word *karuna* means sadness and compassion. How beautiful is that? Compassion is considered the highest form of sadness. It is when someone can really witness someone else's or their own pain and know that we are all dealing with the temporary nature of life. Even the best times must end. There is a real difference between compassion and pity, but they are only separated by a fine line.

Sometimes I would fall to the other side of the line and start to wallow. I'd take a few steps down the road that leads to depression and entertain the thoughts that I had been left behind in Texas. I had to bring myself back. I had to remember that no matter how lonely I felt, this was not Truth. One of the most beautiful truths of life is that we are never truly alone. Sometimes, just when we need it, the perfect person shows up like Lorena did on my first day of work. I have found this to be true many times in life if I can trust the path. We do not have to solve the problem of loneliness, we just have to clear our vision at these moments to see that we are not alone. If we cannot seem to identify a person, we can look to society. There is always someone working to make sure there is food in the grocery store, gas in the pumps, and electricity flowing to our house for us. There is a vast network of support out there with people always crossing paths in mysterious ways. If nothing else, we are always breathing the same air. We are always sharing life with others. The amount of time it took me to cross back over to the side of compassion varied, yet I would always remember that I am not alone. I would remember that my story was not special. This feeling and experience was part of being alive.

It was definitely easier in the long run when I let myself feel. If you can't feel it, you can't heal it became my mantra. I allowed sadness and loneliness to rule my world for an hour or more. Then I would flip the mood. This was a suggestion given to me by Padma that I always followed. It made sure I didn't go to bed deep in the heart of sadness. I'd watch a few short funny videos on my phone, normally cats trying to fit into tiny boxes or wake up their owners, to bring some good hearted laughs. Some warmth would return, and I'd smile as I recalled all I had to be grateful for.

When 90 percent of my YouTube recommendations turned into funny cat videos, I discovered that sometimes, the charm and quirkiness of a cat is all it takes to lift the heaviness of loneliness.

Eighteen

Second Heartbreak

We'd been apart for two years, half of that married, and one day I decided that I'd had enough—our time apart had run its course. We had learned a lot, followed the adventures, and I wanted to see Ryan every day. I updated my resume and started job hunting. I reached out to several people on LinkedIn and asked if they would speak to me about their job or company. Many were more than willing which was really encouraging. I was serious. We were going to be together in California.

After work each day, I looked for openings and applied to several jobs. I remember feeling a strange sense of guilt during this time period. It seemed like I was betraying my current company. I did not like the feeling of saying one thing to them and doing another. I wondered if everyone felt this way when searching for a new job, but I kept moving forward anyway. I started to find roles I liked, but there was always some aspect that made me pause. The company had a recent news scandal, there would be no upward mobility, the commute would not work, and the list went on. That was until I found a job opening at a food manufacturing company with hip, earth-conscious branding. Their products were ones I could get behind, and I knew there was a lot of room to support sustainability in farming, especially in drought-ridden California. I googled the commute and found their office was only five minutes from Ryan's apartment. This opportunity looked promising, so I applied full of anticipation. The next few days I researched further to learn about the company and see if I had any connections for interviews. The online reviews were not stellar. I wished they were better, but that is pretty common. Most people do not rate their company online if they are happily employed. Ryan had reached out to people as well, and found one of our friends from UCLA was close friends with someone who had worked there previously. I was thrilled to know someone with connections, and I thought this could be my chance—until we spoke. She was very open about her experience and did not recommend working there. The culture apparently was less than ideal and she strongly encouraged me to look elsewhere. After hearing her perspective, I knew I could not continue to pursue this lead. I was so disappointed. There certainly would not be another large company near Ryan's apartment.

Shortly after this fall out, Ryan called. "Hey Sarah, I know you may not like this suggestion, but I think you should stay where you are. I think it will be better for you, and I think you will be happier."

"Why?" I asked surprised.

"Because I am nervous you are going to uproot your whole career and then have to do it again when I graduate. You already have a great job, and I may not even be in Los Angeles a lot of the time if you come here. My professor is already talking about me going to DC for the summer," he said.

"I am so tired of the distance," I mentioned.

"I know. Me too. If you were finding lots of jobs you love, then it might be worth considering. But you haven't found something that is a great fit, and I am going to be out of town for at least six months plus traveling to conferences. There is no point in coming here for a job you like less and I'm not home. Plus, you are happy there with your role and yoga."

"Are you really going to be away from Los Angeles for that long?" I asked.

"Yes. At this rate I do not know if other things may come up too. I just wouldn't want you to make such a big move and I am not even here." Ryan had been very successful up to this point. During a six month internship, he created an invention that became a patent. It is nearly unheard of to even identify an idea in that amount of time let alone prove its efficacy. Since returning to UCLA he already had multiple other internship opportunities. These accomplishments did help me start feeling some level of contentment—this path was supporting Ryan's passion and natural talent for science. That was the goal after all.

"Yeah, I hear you," I replied. We decided that night that I would stop job searching. I would stay in Houston until Ryan graduated and was not traveling to different internships. We agreed it made the most sense for both of us. I was in agreement with this decision. I really was. I saw how it actually did not make sense for me to move to Los Angeles at this point. Unfortunately, understanding it logically did not make it less painful. I was so surprised how much this decision hurt. All of the emotions I felt originally resurfaced as if I was back in our hotel room at the Grand Canyon hearing that we would not be together after college. This was my second heartbreak.

I remember feeling so alone that night. I really thought I was going to take action to move to California. I let this idea go as I processed the reality of what was ahead. It's interesting how we can find our voice to set boundaries yet that doesn't necessarily mean things will or should change. We had at least two years if not three more to live long distance. There was still a decent journey ahead. I thought about how it would be nice to talk to someone who had been through this before, but I didn't know anyone—I thought. Then as if my thoughts were being answered, Brittney popped into my mind. How had I almost forgotten that I did know someone who went through the second heartbreak? And a close friend! Brittney, who is also married to her high school sweetheart, had gone through this a few years prior. She and her husband, boyfriend at the time, went to different colleges. When graduation rolled around, we all learned that they had accepted jobs in different states. We were so surprised. When we asked why, we learned Brittney had landed an incredible job in Indiana for her major. It would open so many doors for her career that it would not have made sense to decline. She had gone through the second heartbreak! How did I not realize this sooner? I knew I could use some advice from someone who had walked this trail before. I called Brittney with so much gratitude to once again remember that I am never alone.

Brittney graciously spoke to me for some time when I called. She knew the pain of learning the time would be longer than expected. She ended up leaving her job after one year without another job lined up to end their five years of long distance. And, while I don't remember everything she said, I do recall her telling me, "If I am being honest, I would not recommend quitting your job without having accepted another one. I did it and that was the right thing for me when I did it. We really needed to be back in the same state but it was hard and it's not the best. . . ." And I remember how she empathized with me. I remember feeling seen. I remember feeling understood. Maya Angelou wisely said, "People will forget what you said, people will forget what you did, but people will never forget how you made them feel." I may not remember all her words, but I will always remember that phone call and how she made me feel.

As my heart began to heal from the realization that this journey had many more adventures ahead, I finally began to drop my resistance. The second time around, I began to accept, and I had learned that I must for my health. This was the start of my surrender.

Nineteen

Truth

Shortly after our honeymoon, my supervisor took out a list and placed it on her desk. "These are the five best gastroenterologist doctors in Houston," she said. "Look into them. You need to go to one. I cannot keep seeing you sick like this."

I was very surprised to see she had taken the time to research doctors. With three toddlers of her own at home and ten employees (recent graduates who she often referred to as her work kids) to supervise, she had found time to think about me and take action for me. I had already gone to a gastric doctor who had done a thorough examination so I was not super hopeful this would bring any resolution, but I could not live like this forever, and I was touched by her kindness. I sent the list to my mom and asked if she could help me look into these doctors. She did and scheduled an appointment with the highest-rated one. His office was as far from my house as possible while still being considered Houston. It was almost a two-hour drive which seemed rather inconvenient. I decided to not push back. I would go. The doctor was supposedly very good and my supervisor was offering encouragement.

The first visit ended with the doctor saying I needed to get an endoscopy. I was truly upset by this because I had already gotten an endoscopy that year. Why couldn't they just get the results from the other office? My mom brought me back to earth and reminded me that I would need to do it if I wanted this doctor's evaluation. Fine. I agreed, but if they find nothing this will be the last endoscopy.

My mom flew down for the day of the procedure so I would have someone to drive me home. On the long drive there, I was certainly a little edgy from fasting. I was glad when I was finally in the back room being prepped for the procedure. The anesthesiologist walked through all the last-minute details with me and, because I had been sleeping so poorly, I was excited to be put under. It was guaranteed sleep. It occurred to me that I must be close to rock bottom. So sleep deprived that I was excited about anesthesia. How had my health issues gotten this extreme?

When I woke up, it felt like I had just closed my eyes, so my immediate reaction was disappointment that I couldn't sleep longer until I realized I had no idea how long I'd slept. I looked up to see a nurse at the end of my bed. She reassured me that I may feel a little groggy and I could continue to rest on the bed for now while they got my mom and the doctor reviewed the images. She didn't have to ask me twice to keep resting as I shut my eyes feeling very serene. It wasn't long or maybe it was, I was detached from time from the anesthesia, when we were told the doctor wanted to talk to me and my mom. We sat across the table from the doctor who seemed extremely composed. There was an incredible sense of groundedness and stability to his presence. "The endoscopy went very well," he gently announced. "There was nothing abnormal noted. You have been through some very big changes with graduating college, moving across the country, starting a new job, getting married, and leaving your husband. What you have is . . . anxiety."

His words struck me like a bolt of lightning. Anxiety? I did not have a virus, disease, or physical illness. It was anxiety. It suddenly made sense. I had been trying to use medicine to put out the fire of a broken heart. That was never going to work. A fire needs three things to burn: oxygen, heat, and fuel. It did not matter how many things I had tried to throw at it to snuff out the flames because I was still pouring in the fuel of not accepting my life situation. As long as I was fighting my reality, the flames would keep blazing.

I had not contemplated that I may be experiencing "love sickness," that my emotions were causing this large disturbance. I'm sure my yoga teacher Padma could have told me this all along. She probably instantly saw the root cause was anxiety, but she had the discernment to not tell me because she also saw that I did not yet have the ears to hear it. I needed to sincerely learn how connected thoughts, emotions, and body are for myself. I learned through this challenging experience that they are anything but separate. As I left the doctor's with this diagnosis, I decided that indeed, it was great news. If I was the creator of this madness, I could be the healer of it too.

This is something I can work with, I thought. *It is time to make some changes.*

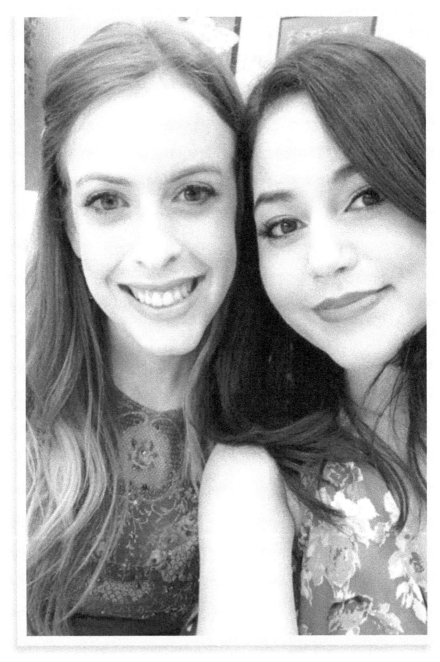

Lorena and I snapped this photo at my bridal shower.
She was a friend I could truly trust in Houston.

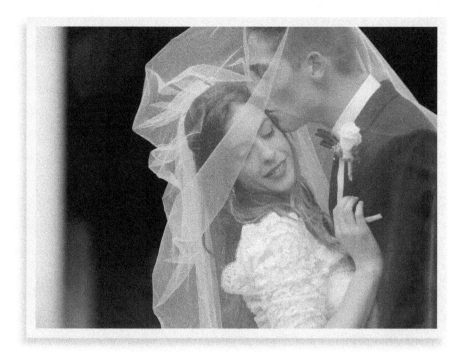

My favorite wedding photo! I always missed Ryan's forehead kisses while we lived apart.

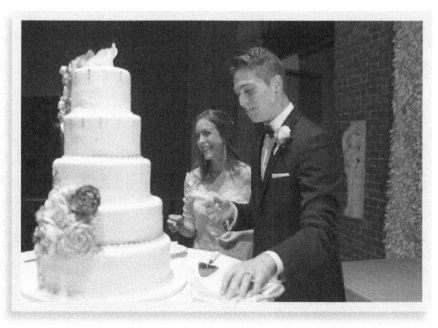

Surprising Ryan after we cut the cake!

Part Three

Healing

What's the point of falling in love if
you both remain inertly as-you-were?

—MARY MCCARTHY, *BETWEEN FRIENDS: THE CORRESPONDENCE OF HANNAH ARENDT AND MARY MCCARTHY, 1949-1975*

My best friend and I ran into German class laughing and out of breath. It was the first day of our freshman year of high school and we clearly had disrupted everyone. We were late because I wanted to try to take a shortcut. My neighbor, who was an upperclassman, showed it to me. She said only the upperclassmen take it and we wanted to be cool. It required going outside which was completely allowed, but it felt rebellious compared to the strict rules of middle school. We were allowed to leave the school doors during school hours? What freedom! Together we trekked outside across school grounds to get to room 110. The school was built in one long line with little pods of about five classrooms each offshooting from the main hall. It reminded me of a photo I had seen in my biology textbook a few days before—a set of lungs with all these little alveolus branching off. All this freedom felt like a breath of fresh air. We made it to our pod and scanned the circle for the room. Our eyes stopped at room 109. Okay, we were close, but where was room 110? A teacher noticed we were lost. "What room are you looking for, dears?"

"We need room 110 with Frau Blauhut," we confidently replied.

"Oh, these are the odd numbered classrooms. The even numbered ones are all the way back on the other side of the school."

There was no way we were going to make it with one minute left. The thought kept running through my mind as to why someone would possibly design a building like this and choose this numbering scheme. We started running without the shortcut this time. At some point along the way we just started laughing and couldn't stop. We were still giggling when we came barreling through the correct door.

This is the first time Ryan ever remembers seeing me. We had been in the same school district with a class size of about two hundred students for eight years, yet our paths had barely crossed. I knew Ryan's name and that he existed, but that was all. Then freshman year we were placed in all the same classes. Much later in the year, he told me that his initial thoughts were, "Who are these random girls who are late on the first day of school?" He definitely judged me and first impressions are important, but luckily I had time to recover from this one.

Twenty

Finding Yoga

"Do you want to come to yoga with me?" my college roommate Elizabeth called to me over her yoga mat clad shoulder, rushing out of the room. "I've been going to the yoga and Pilates classes and they're pretty good, but they aren't at the ritzy SPAC, they are in Patten." The way she lifted her eyebrows when she said SPAC reminded me of how I felt when I walked into the gym on my first tour of Northwestern University while college hunting. The Henry Crown Sports Pavilion, aka SPAC, cardio room was lined with floor to ceiling glass windows that look out over Lake Michigan. Even though I had never done yoga, I thought about what it would feel like to lay my mat out next to one of those windows and breathe deeply, away from the constant hustle of school work, while looking out over the lake. Although it wouldn't be there, I still enthusiastically agreed.

We bundled up in all our winter gear and started out across campus. A snowy mix blew at us as we walked faster, backs hunched over, doing our best to block our faces from the great lake's wind. I had never been to the Patten gym as it was mainly used for intramural sports. My first impression as I walked in was gratitude for the warmth of the heat on my skin, and secondly, I couldn't help but take in the Old English Men's Club vibe that was reflected in the dark wooden stairs and mahogany lined windows. It seemed like an unlikely place to find my zen but my friend signaled for me to follow her up the stairs as she walked to a dimly lit back room that seemed fairly tucked away. The atmosphere was not my preferred type of decor, but I was curious what this would be like. I had no real attachment to if I was going to like the class and was happy to simply spend some time with my roommate. As an engineering major, most of my friends were guys, and I craved more time with my girlfriends because I knew I needed more of that feminine energy in my day. After a quick perusal of the space, Elizabeth and I chose two spots closest to the back and unrolled our mats. I felt a slight nervousness move over my body while I waited for the instructor to begin the class. After a brief moment of silence and then intention setting (mine was to just get through the class without thinking of the pile of work waiting for me back at my room!), we were directed to move through a sun salutation: cobra, head lifted to the sky, a nice big bend in our backs, to down dog where we were instructed to get our heels as close to the floor as possible. After that we flowed into triangle pose, and as I stared at my left hand, reaching for the sun, I noticed a miracle that nearly knocked me off my feet. For the first time in weeks, my heart was beating at a slow and steady pace and didn't feel like it was going to rip right through my chest! I relished in the calm and reflected over the events of that afternoon as I moved into child's pose, pressing my third eye squarely into the middle of the mat. In my mind's eye, I could see myself sitting there that morning, knowing I needed to be concentrating on the professor's lecture, but instead, overwhelmed and distracted with counting the thumping of my heart inside my rib cage. My massive heart arrhythmia, unbeknownst to my differential equations professor, made evident by all the scratching of equations he continued to perform on the board at the front of the room, was madness. As he began to list our homework for the week with the tiny piece of chalk he had left from all the derivatives and integrals, my heart beat faster. My stress had been escalating to an abnormal level this semester as differential equations, mass and energy balance, organic chemistry, and US environmental policy all threatened to take over my sanity.

Even through all my angst, I had actually come to love organic chemistry. It was the first course of chemical engineering that actually involved chemistry. Unfortunately, liking it didn't lessen the number of hours it took to study and master the discipline. I looked around the room, hoping I could find proof that I was not the only one who was feeling completely overwhelmed. I felt a passing twinge of relief when I could feel the same tension radiating off the student next to me. Her lips were pursed and her eyes bugged out with each passing item our professor listed as due. "She probably has a perfectionist issue like me," I thought as I scrambled to copy every due date down in my planner. My assumption that I wasn't the only one who felt the assignments were nearly impossible to handle turned out to be correct; fifty percent of our class would drop out after that initiation, leaving the other half of us to suffer with our equations and impossible deadlines. As I moved through another downward dog sequence, I realized that I finally felt a sense of calm, for the first time in weeks. And I wanted more.

I attended yoga classes for the entire semester and gradually noticed it was the only hour in my entire week where my heart slowed down and beat at a natural rhythm, instead of beating like a gong inside my chest. It was such a relief to have found a moment of peace. As I moved through sequence after sequence I couldn't help but wonder: Could this systematic method be part of the equation to the happiness

I was seeking? I wasn't sure I had that answer, but I felt an immediate connection to yoga and knew there was more I needed to learn about it. If just one hour could make such a potent impact, there had to be more peace to be found to fill my days.

I had been lucky enough to have the opportunity to intern at several companies around the country during college and it was in the middle of one of these internships that I discovered my first yoga studio. This was a revelation to me; that there were spaces dedicated for this practice was mind blowing and exciting. I had not considered that there were businesses that specialized in teaching yoga outside of gyms. The atmosphere was so much more serene, what with their intentional color schemes, essential oil fragrances wafting in to meet you when you walked through the door. The soothing sounds of pan flutes and chimes instantly brought ease and relaxation to my body as soon as I heard it. I discovered they offered an expansive array of levels and the teachers had more in-depth training than the classes I had taken at the school gym. During one internship in Baton Rouge, Louisiana, I visited a yoga studio every night for the full three months I was in town. This brought to life for me that yoga not only incorporated physical strength, flexibility, and balance, but also mental and emotional stability. I *loved* how much it encompassed! At first this was because it fulfilled my need for efficiency.

For as long as I can remember, I had always felt like I didn't have enough time. I had an insatiable desire to experience life and could never comprehend why anyone would waste their time when life is short and there is so much possibility. My passions and ambitions continually led me to have thoughts like: *There is not enough time each day! . . . Life is too short! . . . Is a lifetime long enough for all I want to see and create?*

. . . How can I fit the most into each day? So much so that I would say thoughts out loud, and in high school, Ryan bought me a rose quartz crystal bracelet with the engraving *Time is Precious*. I definitely felt seen. I cherished that bracelet and it became my constant reminder to never waste a moment. Now I was feeling that yoga could allow me to achieve many benefits in one practice versus needing several different forms of exercise and hobbies to be well rounded. I sensed yoga could be transformative even beyond this integration, but in the various states I had lived, I had only been able to find places that taught the physical aspect with some minor meditation dispersed in here and there. When I decided to learn more about yoga, I asked a teacher I met in Maine what she recommended. She advised me to purchase three versions of the *Yoga-sutras* of Patanjali and look for my answers there. She explained that reading several versions is important because there is no perfect translation from Sanskrit and by reading various translations, I could more closely interpret the original message. I, of course, did exactly as she said. My perfectionist tendencies would follow me everywhere! I poured over the hefty text in my free time and it filled me with joy. I began to underline everything I felt was important and applied myself as I tried to understand this vast, ancient philosophy that I had so many questions about. I most remember feeling overwhelmed by the concept of *mind*. There were so many words and nuances just for the mind: *manas, citta, buddhi,* and *ahamkara.* The many concepts presented in the sutras brought back memories of overflowing equations on my professor's chalkboard, but instead of being filled with fear and anxiety, I was filled with curiosity. I was enthusiastic to study and dissect every equation even if I did not understand everything I read. For the first time, perhaps in my entire life, I was content to have open and unanswered questions. Large portions of a snow day would be spent under a cozy blanket underlining sentences that spoke to me and contemplating what it all meant. I turned each page with care and

relished the opportunity to learn—at my own pace, without deadlines, for my own development, by my choice, with no final grade. It was so freeing, my body felt weightless. A passion to learn carried me forward and led me to continue to read despite the tedious nature of interpreting lessons that are meant to be conveyed by a teacher. I took copious notes and filled a notebook with the main takeaways from every sutra. It took me months to finish reading the first copy and my curiosity was piqued, especially since I only understood about 30 percent of the text. I later learned that I started off reading one of the hardest translations of the *Yoga-sutras*, but I am grateful because having trouble comprehending the sutras and only understanding 30 percent of the text increased my desire to find a yoga teacher who could help me understand the other 70 percent. I truly wanted to learn about all eight limbs of yoga and not solely the physical postures, since it was clear to me that this part had to be integrated into one's life to find peace. I sensed this knowledge held a key for me, on how to be happy, and I was eager to do whatever was needed in order to find out. I didn't know how I was going to do it, a Midwestern engineering student at the young age of twenty-one, but I was convinced there was a way to learn the full picture of yoga.

My first clue had arrived when the random yogini in Louisiana recommended I take a teacher training course, which I had taken to heart, but that was going to be two years after college. So until then, I needed to find a teacher who could guide me. I now had a lot of conviction, but I had no idea how to find a teacher. Previously, I had taken classes with an advanced yogi who clearly seemed to know the practice beyond the postures from a guru. I was so impressed every time I saw him. He had a collected, calm, and in charge presence about him. I will always recall him sitting in the front of class with his legs perfectly crossed in lotus pose saying, "You may hear some teachers say, choose your intention for being in class. The intention for all yoga classes is to find enlightenment. That is always the intention. You do not need to choose an intention beyond self-realization." His tone was firm, yet without judgment. His presence was always an embodiment of what yoga is really about—I felt that if anyone knew how to find a guru, it would be him. After one of his classes, I finally gathered the courage to ask him, "How did you find your guru?"

He had his right shoulder turned toward me and without even turning to fully face me he simply looked in my direction, skirted my question and said, "When the student is ready, the teacher will appear." I was crestfallen—I thought it would be more straightforward than that. I decided to change tactics, and nervously shifted from one bare foot to the other. I desperately wanted to know beyond this common yoga phrase, which is often repeated. I cleared my throat and asked again, with more specificity this time, "Well, how and when did you find your guru?"

He replied with a small grin and the same shrug and repeated his first answer: "When the student is ready, the teacher will appear." His energy conveyed that it was not a question that could be asked and simply answered. His path was his path and my path was going to be mine. This was not like getting trained for another work position. This was a specific life calling. I was going to have to find a teacher on my own. Even with the non-answer answer, there was a passion that had been ignited inside me, and I was going to be ready.

Twenty-One

Rasa Yoga

The room was so hot, the thermometer registered at ninety-eight degrees, which was even hotter than it was out in the Houston sun and which I definitely had not adjusted to in the four days since my move there. Sweat kept dripping from my hair line into my right eye and I was afraid I was going to slip off my mat, right on top of the dumbbells I had laid out for the next part of the class. Outstretched in extended side angle, the teacher instructed us to grab the weights from our mat and complete five bicep curls. Even though the teacher really seemed to have a beautiful energy about him, his proclamation at the beginning of the class about this being the studio's signature class, was enough for me to know I needed to find another place to practice. The class was intriguing, and while I loved the physical challenge, I was searching for traditional yoga and I had a deep hunger to learn the depths of yoga philosophy. This was one of the main reasons I felt drawn to California; I knew there were so many accomplished yogis to learn from. Sighing heavily as the class ended, I dropped my dumbbells back into a bin, knowing this would be the last time I would come here. I was ready to learn, not simply work out. As I packed up my mat and water bottle, I made a commitment to myself to keep searching for the right place. It had to be out there.

The Houston suburbs were a beautiful area, filled with manicured lawns and upscale shopping malls that offered anything money could buy. But, I realized even before moving there that I might have to commute to downtown Houston, a much more diverse and urbanized area, to find the heart-centered traditional yoga training that I was craving. I was fully prepared to do that, but I still wanted a local spot where I could take classes on the weekdays. I rolled up my mat in resignation, and headed for the door, and as I was just about to walk through the threshold, the owner blocked my way.

"How did you like the class?" His eyes locked directly onto mine, and he was just so sincere. I hesitated and fiddled with my mat. I didn't know how honest I should be—he was so caring, I didn't want to hurt his feelings. I diverted the conversation and shared that I was new to the area and on the hunt for my yoga home. He handed me a flier for an event called the Bay Area Yoga Collective for the next Saturday. "All the local yoga studios will be there offering free classes with the owners," he explained excitedly. I felt hope start to replace the disappointment and defeat I was carrying out of the yoga studio as I enthusiastically accepted the invitation, relaxing in the comfort that the Universe had provided for me, and so quickly. As I walked to my car, I couldn't wait for the next week to roll around. I didn't know it yet, but I had just been handed my ticket to my guru. I had known nothing about finding a yoga teacher, even though I thought I knew all the right places to search, but luckily, I was apparently ready as a student, because my guru would finally appear in the suburbs of Houston only fifteen minutes away from my cousin's house.

———

Strolling into the park for the Bay Area Yoga Collective with my head held high, I was overjoyed to see so many people walking in with their yoga mats slung over their shoulders. It was a festive occasion with local vendor booths surrounding the pavilion selling all the organic, free trade goodies yogis would naturally buy. Right at the entrance was the Rasa Yoga booth and it couldn't be missed, what with one of their teachers spinning around nearly upside down on a pole they had brought from their pole studio. In the background was a large, colorful wheel off to the side of the display table, where they were enthusiastically inviting people up to spin the wheel to see what they would win. The teacher slid down the pole as he saw me walk closer.

"Hey come on up! Try your hand at spinning the wheel!" I giggled because if there is anything I love, it's a raffle. I love winning and I have quite good raffle karma. "Have you heard of us?" he asked as I took my turn and spun the wheel with all my might.

I looked at him with confusion when he said us. "I mean Rasa Yoga."

"Oh, no, I am new to the area." Before I knew it, I had a consultation appointment for the next Monday to see the studio. His authentic, open energy had an allure that made me want to see what else this place had to offer. When I walked in the doors that Monday for the first time, I immediately loved the serene yet vibrant atmosphere of Rasa Yoga. All the rooms were so colorful in an elegant way that showed every aspect had been thought out with love. I was greeted by another caring teacher who offered me some hot tea and guided me through their various classes and advanced trainings that were available. I was so surprised to learn that they offered a comprehensive curriculum centered around yoga philosophy. It was even called a yoga school instead of a yoga studio because education was the main focus. The space was everything I had been imagining while searching for a space, and I could feel the authenticity radiate right into my heart, from everyone I met. I certainly wanted to return yet I won't say it was love at first sight. When I was offered an introductory discount on three months of tuition if I signed up that evening, I declined with hesitation. Three months was a long time if this turned out to not be the place for me, and although I wouldn't bat an eye at the amount it cost now, right out of college, it seemed like a large investment. In my hesitation, I didn't know that what I had stepped into was so massive that I could not see the full view of how aligned the school was with what I had been seeking. The offerings at the school were just too extensive to be introduced to in an instance. As time unfolded, I would understand that I had found the community my heart had yearned for and one of the best yoga schools in America.

When I went home that evening, I didn't feel settled. My agitation grew until I realized that the three months was a small risk to see if I had found my yoga home, so I called back really late that same evening asking if they would let me sign up for the three months over the phone. A few hours of space had brought me clarity, and it still astonishes me that anyone even answered my call at that hour. But then again, unusual occurrences certainly ensue when something is our calling.

A few months into taking classes at Rasa Yoga, I finally met the founder Padma Shakti, which I had been anxiously awaiting. She was leading a workshop on the idea of prosperity. I had a hunger to know the founder of this yoga school that offered education on all aspects of yoga; I wanted to know how she had come to possess this knowledge. This workshop was a six-week series based around a book. We were assigned chapters to read each week, and invited to answer the reflection questions at the end. Throughout the course, I kept a list of questions I wanted to ask Padma, if I ever had the opportunity. Most of them were not appropriate to ask during the workshop because they were not about the workshop, but I was hopeful I would get a chance someday.

I did finally muster the courage to ask a question when I returned my focus to the actual workshop topic: "I hear what you are saying, but what if you can't change something in your life?" Her reply is a lesson I will never forget.

"Can I offer you something around your wording to that question?" Padma asked with a gentle directness.

Of course I was open to hearing. I had been waiting to speak with and meet the owner herself, someone I barely knew but already sensed I admired, and I was eager to hear her feedback. I didn't perceive this question as being corrected but simply feedback to help me gain more insight. I've learned from having many coaches in my life that no matter how painful, feedback always supports me in the long run. Padma proceeded to open my eyes. "Try to avoid the words *I can* and *I can't*, and instead replace them with *I am willing* or *I am not willing*. Like if someone asks you to go to dinner and you say you can't, that is probably not true. It just is not a priority. Or when someone tells me they cannot come to yoga for this or that reason, it normally is just not a priority for them. Most of the time, we can make it to things, if it is our priority. If it is not, be truthful and certain in your answer. Try, instead, to say I am willing or not willing. Then, and only then, are you being honest with yourself, and with others," she stated.

This was quite a perspective shift for me and it brought up some butterflies in my stomach, a feeling I would get used to as I studied more yoga and faced old patterns. As I contemplated these words for the next few weeks, I perceived the truth in it right away, and also felt the contraction of how this would require some courage to implement in certain areas of my life. In true guru fashion, Padma had shed light on a pattern that was not serving me to expand my self-awareness in our first very short but poignant interaction. As I pondered the motive behind my willingness to attend something or help someone, I changed my vocabulary and stopped myself whenever I felt like responding to someone with "I can't." For example, something I really wanted was to make new friends in my new home city of Houston. In order to make those new friends, I was willing to drive forty minutes to meet those people in an effort to connect. What I wasn't willing to do (instead of saying I can't) was go to happy hour every weekend and drink alcohol as soon as the clock struck 4:00 p.m. It was the first of many small lessons I would learn that would require me to take responsibility for my own life. Many of these small lessons, over time, would start to guide me down the path where I was willing and able to accept my reality. When I truly honored that I was not doing something because it was not a priority, then I could no longer be a victim in the situation. I was in charge of making the decisions that created my life.

With more emotionally charged situations, the places in my life where I had previously considered I was the victim were not always pleasant to see. For example, the emotionally charged situation of wanting to be with Ryan. What was I willing to choose in order to make that happen? Well, I was willing to fly often from Houston to LA and brainstorm with him ideas for the future. However, I was not willing to change jobs right after college in order to do that. After a lot of self-reflection, I realized it was also a priority for me to not burn bridges or look flakey on my resume.

Hard Truth. I wanted my life to be with Ryan, but I also wanted other things too.

I learned when I was willing to see these hard truths, healing could begin. I needed to learn how to come back to myself and be honest about how I wanted to shape my life. My situation was forcing me to play small or strengthen my character. I had always been with Ryan which was wonderful, but I had to face this rite of passage to learn how to stand firmly on my own. And the long journey to healing had begun. Me, and only me, was responsible for my life.

I had found my guru. Suddenly I knew why I had decided to come to Texas.

Twenty-Two

Change in Consciousness

My yoga mentor Gracie often references this quote from Albert Einstein when she teaches how important perspective is to maneuver to a new level in life: "You cannot solve a problem with the same consciousness that created it." This is very much where I was at after having been told the truth by the gastroenterologist. I had anxiety—plain and simple. I reflected back on my H. pylori research and recalled how in one thread on the internet where someone was seeking advice for my same symptoms there was a single reply out of hundreds where a man wrote, "You are not going to want to hear this, but your issue is anxiety and my grandmother went through this same experience." He was completely dismissed while all the other suggestions had comments and replies. I remember his reply so vividly, and although it made an impression on me, I, too, dismissed it without merit while thinking his grandmother and I likely didn't have the same issue—never looking into his suggestion further. Now, after hearing it from a reputable doctor, I was ready and able to listen. After providing me with this diagnosis, the gastric doctor further elaborated that trauma had caused some valve along my esophagus to stay permanently open when it should open and close while eating. He told me to take an anxiety medication for one month. The medicine would relax the valve so it would remember its natural muscle memory, and I would not need the medicine after the month was over. He was very clear that this medicine was not addictive which helped put me at ease. Within two days of taking the pills, all the burping had stopped, and the nonstop internal torture I had been experiencing in my esophagus for over a year was gone. It was miraculous. Finally, I could breathe. I could think. I could eat.

I already believed the diagnosis, but after the pills worked so well, there was no doubt as to the root cause of my symptoms. It was time to change my consciousness so I could solve my problems. My perspective started to shift the instant I heard his prognosis. I was not a victim. In fact, I was empowered because I understood what I was experiencing; *dis*-ease. And it was clearly time to find *ease*. My body had been screaming at me, begging for help this entire time, but I didn't know how to listen. Now I knew I had the ability to choose how I was going to proceed forward. I flipped back open my *The Secret of the Yoga Sutra* book by Pandit Rajmani Tigunait and read the first sutra, a natural place to start. *Atha yoganusasanam*: Now begins the instruction of the practice of yoga. It implies that whenever the sutras cross your path in life, now is the time to begin yoga. Atha translates to *now*, and also an auspicious beginning where your journey has prepared you for the road ahead. The time to start is now, atha.

My first small step was setting up an appointment at the salon. I had kept my hair long for my big day, so I could have luscious, flowing curls with my wedding dress but it had been weighing me down. It was too time consuming to professionally style all that hair before work each morning. As I walked in, I got a whiff of the familiar smell of hairspray and essential oils. My hairdresser, Padma's talented daughter, signaled for me to come over and sit in the chair. I was so eager to make a drastic shift as I enthusiastically showed her how much of my long locks I wanted to chop off by pointing to a line at my shoulders. "Well, we don't need to shampoo all this hair if we are cutting that much off," she said as she grabbed a hair tie and proceeded to put my hair in a ponytail. "I'm going to cut right here and then we'll style it—you're sure you're ready?" I nodded yes and then my ponytail was gone. I relished in the head massage, inarguably the best part of any haircut, while she shampooed what hair was left and released tension held in my scalp. My hair hadn't been this short since I was six, which I only knew from seeing photos in family albums. It was like letting go of the past and returning to my past, simultaneously. This was one of the simplest changes I made yet it felt so symbolic. My head felt light and free, and my past lay on the floor beneath me. There were new things waiting up ahead.

After making significant adjustments, I continued to assess where I most needed a shift in my life. I had been experiencing low back pain for about five years, and this stood out as a large factor that needed to be addressed. I had tried many remedies, every medical profession available and nothing had panned out. I had done years of physical therapy, acupuncture, chiropractic work, neuromuscular therapy, and still, no relief. Finally, I decided to take private yoga classes with the therapists at Rasa Yoga because, like my stomach problem, I wanted to find the root cause of the pain. I had been hesitant to try, honestly I had given up hope for a cure, but it was absolutely worth trying because my back pain was limiting me. I'll always remember sitting on my mat in the middle of the studio for my first session with Gracie and Denise, both advanced therapists at Rasa Yoga, across from me. I felt so small in the large room without other students, so it did somewhat help to have two yoga therapists to fill the room. Normally, there would be one but Denise was finishing up training of her own so Gracie was also there to observe. I kept repeatedly reading the painted words on the walls while I waited for the lesson to start—Sustainability, Fun, Desire, Power, Passion, Community—as if they could provide me the answers I needed for whatever Gracie and Denise may ask of me. My body was still but inside my mind was fidgeting with nerves from the personalized attention I was about to receive from two people I looked up to. I was simultaneously giddy from feeling a spark of hope for the first time in a long time about my back. The lesson started by Denise asking me the natural questions of what my intention for lessons was and what I hoped to gain from our time. I provided my backstory around sciatica pain and somewhat quietly stated, "I want to know how to support my back and learn the correct pelvic position for every orientation: standing, sitting, lying on my back, lateral movements, and twists." Her eyebrows lifted, lips pursed, and head tilted, giving all the tell-tale signs that she was surprised with how precise I was in my answer. After a breath, she reassured me that she could teach me all of this. A few sessions later I was balancing in warrior three with my leg out behind me when I heard Denise once again say, "Navel center—focus on your navel center. You're sinking into your lower back again." I had lost count of how many times I had been told this. It had become clear that a lot of my pain was caused from overworking my back muscles because I was sinking into my lower back from not engaging my core. Philosophically, I had learned, this is a sign of giving away my power and linked to the third chakra. Everything was beginning to come full circle. To heal, I needed to relearn how to walk, stand, and exercise to avoid putting pressure on my low back and reclaim my worth. Every second I was conscious, I had to ask myself, "Am I using my core? How do I need to adjust my posture?" I found that healing often requires a tedious, nonstop journey of mastering the fundamentals. I literally went all the way back to relearning how to walk, to experience a physical relearning which in turn reprogrammed my mental and spiritual faculties. The mind and body are intricately interwoven. It was a long and slow journey, and these times force us to honestly ask ourselves the question, *How much do I really want to heal?*

My answer this time, like the past, was *very much*. I was willing to go back to the very beginning if that is what it took. Over time I saw significant improvement, but there were times when my old patterns would resurface. The pain would return and I would want to collapse on the floor and return to wallowing in my sorrow. It was hard work to sustain that level of presence from how I was walking to how I was sleeping. During one of these relapses, I remember meeting with Gracie. She asked me, "What if you always have this back pain?" I was not sure I understood the question. Always have this back pain? How could that be an option? She knew exactly what I was thinking in the silence between her question and what she said next. "Can you accept the reality that you may deal with this your whole life? I do not mean to stop trying to heal it. You can continue to work toward and envision it being healed. At the same time, can you find peace with it being lifelong?" I felt a heaviness in my heart that I sighed out as I gazed out the window. I saw the sidewalk I walked up every day and considered whether I wanted to keep walking in the door with the majority of my thoughts being about my back. I was starting to get it. Could I find peace along the journey with no attachment to the end result? This concept she presented was powerful. And as I mulled it over, considered it, reflected on it and held this truth in my hands, I could see that it was the key to shifting my relationship with my back. Gracie was trying to teach me how to be truly content, or *santosha,* a vital component of the second limb of yoga. Could I accept this reality in its entirety? Could I accept that healing cannot be accomplished through achievement? If this was how my back was always going to be, could I be content with life, even with this pain? I was ready for this lesson because Gracie asked me to study contentment before. For an entire year, I had made santosha my word of the year and reflected on how this is experienced through the lens of each of my week's events. On a daily basis I considered whether I could be content to do nothing for a day, or whether I could be content with the present moment without changing anything? Now she was waking me up to the next question: Could I be content to live with this pain? I was transported to a memory of another therapy session where she and Denise were guiding me on healing my back. Goddess pose started to make me shake and as I adjusted my back, other alignment points moved, causing me to start questioning myself and if I could ever correct my posture. I cannot recall the exact words Denise used, but she looked up at me with curious eyes and said, "You are so smart, talented, kind, successful, courageous, beautiful, and compassionate. But do you see that? Why do you question yourself?" I felt authenticity and tender love in her words. Emotion welled up inside of me as warmth moved immediately up my spine into my heart. Still, I wanted to be perceived as strong, so I did not let the tears surface. I wish I had because the flow of those tears would have likely washed away so much pain that was lodged deep inside me. In that moment, my pride stopped the healing from fully arising, but that didn't mean I didn't hear her words. As I continued through the session, I wondered why I didn't lead with seeing myself this way. Why did I not see myself as enough? When was I going to be enough? Was there a situation where I would accept that I am already enough? Standing back beside Gracie, I understood there was no perfect endpoint. Could I be content and accept myself in the now, in all my beauty, flaws, and pain? Yes. I could. I had to, because that was the only way to heal. That night, I accepted my pain. I found she had the same voice as me and was trying to help me all along. We became friends and spoke often. I would remind myself that I am enough as many times as it took. This brought significant peace into my life.

It was not lost on me that this same concept could be applied to my relationship with Ryan and I being apart. This one was much harder for me to be content with, and although it took more time, I was beginning to open the door of acceptance.

Within a few months, I shifted the landscape of my life dramatically. Looking back, I see the irony in that even my last name changed after our wedding. Not only had my environment changed, but also my identity, literally.

New job. New hair. New address. New name. New license plates. New outlook.

I was ready to be at ease.

Twenty-Three

Sing and Dance

Wind whisked through my hair, whispering that all would be okay as I sat on the gazebo's wooden bench. The gazebo was around the corner from the home I rented after our wedding on the edge of the Gulf of Mexico with its vast expanse of bluish gray waters. It had become a favorite spot of mine to decompress and gaze out over all the jumping fish constantly flying out of the water. Occasionally I would walk far out onto the precarious looking dock and swing my legs over the edge mesmerized by the vastness of the ocean. Sometimes, on hard days, I would even drive home during my lunch break to eat at the gazebo to remember the broader world around me. This Sunday morning I had allowed myself a break from my overly motivated to-do list and was basking in the stillness with a new book. Feeling the weight of a new story in my hands brought joy and anticipation as I flipped to the first page. The journey had just begun when I spotted a man in his late fifties in my peripheral vision wearing a plain white T-shirt and loose athletic shorts. Casually, swaying to his own tune, he hummed all the way to the waterline with his head held high in a soft smile. Humming switched to singing when he turned to walk toward the gazebo still lost in song.

His eyes looked up as his left foot touched the first stair landing. "Oh! I thought I was out here alone. I hope I wasn't bothering you there. I just came out here to sing. I believe God just wants us to sing and dance, even if we aren't good at it. I believe that makes God smile, so I just come out here to sing."

He then graciously kept walking by as he sang from his heart to let me be at the gazebo alone. It was a brief, bizarre encounter that oddly felt magical. Who was he? I had never seen him in the neighborhood before and would never see him again, yet he seemed so at ease in this space. I sensed even more grace in his soul when he had the wherewithal to perceive that I needed a quiet morning and kept walking by without a moment of hesitation. His energy was somewhat akin to the innocence of a child and I was transported back to an evening at my cousin's house when I was still quite sick my first year after college. I was sitting at the living room table doing some work with the little energy left that I could muster. As I typed a response to an email for work, I heard the beep of my cousin's SUV followed by the familiar click of the gate signaling that she and Raylan were home as they rounded the corner to the house. As she opened the door I heard, "Hey Pretzel, we have a request for you!" in a happy and slightly higher tone than normal. I couldn't imagine what it could possibly be. I remember my first thought being, *I am so burned out, will I be able to do the request?*

"Hey, I am over here," I replied. "What is it?"

"Hey! Raylan has been asking to dance with you the entire ride home. I do not know why, but that is all he wants."

As I rounded the corner to the kitchen, Raylan bent his knees to get real low, grinned as wide as his little face would let him and yelled, "Pretzel, pretzel come dance with me!" His nickname for me always was endearing and I nodded yes to him so relieved that this was a request I could do. "Outside Pretzel. Over here!" Raylan signaled for me to step outside on the porch and he took my hands and started jumping. We were both just jumping up and down together with both hands clasped. "We're dancing, we're dancing!" he exclaimed with the biggest smile I had ever seen. It was quite adorable—my smile quickly became as big as his and my cousin started filming because it was such a profound moment. By the end we were all bursting out with laughter taking in the moment of spontaneous "dancing" that Raylan had prescribed for us. We laughed so much that all of our bellies hurt. Sweetness oozed out of Raylan and he brought us all joy. He always knew just what was needed, and that night, it was a short dance party.

That dance party brought life back into my soul on a difficult day. The man's words at the gazebo had brought back a precious memory and he grabbed my attention in an expansive way. I felt I was being asked to hear his message. It was a message I recognized beyond jumping without a care in the world. One I had heard before. Bhakti yoga is a devotional branch of yoga that uses dancing and singing to find universal consciousness, oftentimes chanting and dancing from dusk to dawn lost in the joy of it all. Many stories are told that when a devotee is singing and dancing there is no more devotee—they become absorbed in the dance. In other words, they are no longer their ego and have merged into the oneness of life that connects us all. It is akin to whirling dervishes, like the poet Rumi, who believe that getting lost in dance and song is a spiritual discipline for your soul. There are many paths and cultures with similar philosophies. Knowing this, it just seemed so strange for someone to walk by singing, tell me that, and keep walking by. How many people would keep walking and allow me to have my alone time with the water and jumping fish? It was unexpected to say the least. I interpreted it as a sacred Sunday synchronicity that I would take to heart; validation even for allowing myself to enjoy what I love that morning on the rickety bench.

I reflected on what I could learn here. Was I taking life too seriously? Did I need to let my hair down and dance to my favorite song? Could I be taking healing too seriously? And could healing really be that simple?

It's ironic how the simplest of things can feel so hard. Why does fear take such a strong hold when we try to trust and let go?

I closed my eyes to hear the message again; this loving tone was all I needed to move through these questions, gradually loosen my grip, and dance to my inner song.

Twenty-Four

Konnichiwa

Before one of our phone calls, Ryan let me know by text that he had a big update to discuss that night. I recall being so curious as to what he had to tell me because he's the type to only send a cryptic text if the news is significant.

"Hey, so I wanted to talk to you about this the next time you visited, but it sounds like I may need to decide sooner than I thought. My professor mentioned he may have an opportunity for me to work in Japan. Obviously that is a pretty big commitment and we would be further apart, so I wanted to talk it over with you."

My heart skipped a beat when I heard his news. While I wasn't overly jazzed about being an ocean apart now, I did notice this small spark of excitement inside me, and I was surprised. "Wow, that is a big opportunity. How long would you be in Japan?" I asked. There was a brief silence on the other end of the phone. The hesitation got me wondering if he was going to say years.

"It would be for six months," he confessed. My immediate thought was that of course he needed to go! These are the opportunities you don't pass up in life—this is what he had been working toward. I'd experienced how good it could be when one moved through life with a *yes* mentality. I wanted Ryan to walk through all the open doors available to him. But I was conflicted. I would miss him desperately, I knew this distance in our meetups would cause an ache inside me I didn't want to experience. But the other part, I realized as I listened to him describe the details of this opportunity, was that I didn't want to be left behind. I wanted to drop my life and see Japan too! We had spoken many times about living abroad and decided that if one of our jobs presented the chance, we would enjoy living out of the country for a year or two. I had imagined it in all of my dreams of our life together. This door flew open faster than I anticipated and my life was not in a place to drop everything and move to Japan. I did contemplate this, though, and imagined myself leading with complete spontaneity and abandonment—until I considered the reality that neither one of us would have a job after six months and a home mortgage to pay. I honestly told Ryan how I was feeling and that my main heartache was that I wanted to move there, too, and experience this incredible life moment together. I felt sad about the prospect of not sharing another new life adventure. He empathized long enough for me to know I had to shift my perspective and be grateful that I would get to visit and experience a new culture because of this amazing opportunity. He let me know the chance of him going, if he was willing, was essentially guaranteed. As I hung up the phone, I started processing this life change. Our relationship was about to go from being long distance to *longer* distance.

Over the next few months, the details started to solidify; Ryan would be flying to Japan in September. I desperately wanted to be there that first week and get to live somewhere versus visit as a tourist. So I spent time contemplating how I could be there. I reviewed the time I had off and the company policies and finally let Ryan know that I wanted to come for an entire month, which would require that I request two weeks unpaid time off. I think he was surprised by my bold proposal. He wanted to see me, but he was concerned. He did not want me to jeopardize my work relationships and was worried I would be bored if he was working all day in a country where I didn't speak the language. Leaving for a month was definitely not normal for the company culture. I, of course, did not know what the implications would be, but I knew this was a once in a lifetime opportunity. I would have regrets if I did not try to visit for a long enough time to really see Japan and get a glimpse into what it is like to live there. My mind was made up.

It was quite scary to ask for a month off and for half of that to be unpaid. I really had to face my fears of being told no and being judged as a less-serious employee. It was so programmed into me that any difference between me and the other employees would lead to poor evaluations and being passed by for promotions that it rendered me feeling close to powerless. I was lacking in life experience; the kind that would show me I could always get another job if a company didn't value me and that I was even capable of generating my own revenue. Something I now know but was so unfamiliar to me then that I would walk on eggshells if that was the requested rule. This outlook required me to chip away at my fear—literally crack through my shell of doubt—to step onto smoother terrain. I recalled all the lessons from Padma on owning my self-worth and to never forget my brilliance. I needed to let my higher, expanded self who could create my world lead. My yoga training certainly contributed to me trusting that this really could happen if I just asked, and I deeply felt it was a risk worth taking. The more I trained, the stronger my voice grew which is related to the concept of *udan vayu*, an upward movement in the body associated with exhalation and expression. Yoga practices help strengthen udan vayu to give rise to the ability to speak your Truth and set boundaries, valuable lessons for me. Japan was another opportunity to practice using my udan vayu. I had gotten to where I had told everyone in my life except for my supervisor who could actually make the decision. Then one morning courage called me forward in the form of a trusted coworker with a cute blonde pixie cut. She strutted toward me grinning, practically giggling, and blurted out because she couldn't keep it in anymore, "She is in a really good mood today! You need to go ask for that time off now! Go now! I'm serious." When I didn't immediately walk toward our supervisor's door, my coworker continued to encourage me that this was the moment. She was giving me serious now-or-never energy, so I leaned into trust and called on courage as I walked into my supervisor's office on the spot, without notice, and asked for time off with no pay. My coworker didn't lead me astray. Our supervisor was not just in a good mood but an *excellent* mood and I got instant approval. There were some sticky moments down the road but I got what I wanted because I leaned into my own heart . . . and as my mom taught me, anticipation is always worse than the actual event. When it came time for me to actually leave for Japan, it was a big deal in the office. Everyone was amazed that someone had figured out how to leave for a month. Everyone said the same thing when they found out: "Is that even possible?" Many of the younger employees were curious how I had pulled it off.

———————

With my trip to Japan set, I chose to allocate my other vacation days for the year differently since I would see Ryan for so long at the end of the year. I decided I was going to go on the eleven-day yoga retreat taking place in Austin, Texas, that was part of my teacher training certification. I thought it was not going to be possible while we were long distance and now it was happening. I couldn't wait to walk the fields among the peacocks! Life is full of surprises and it was shaping up to be a great year.

Twenty-Five

Heard

I looked down at my phone and read the text. "We had to close the heat exchanger. They needed to get on to the next job." Heat exchangers are critical to the operation of any chemical unit as they help heat up the chemical feed so that it is hot enough to create whichever reaction you are performing. One of ours was being cleaned, which is done sparingly to improve profits, so it is important to inspect the insides for any damage that may need to be repaired before it is sealed back up, potentially for years. Anger rose inside me as I reread the message. This was another attempt to ensure I could not do my job or even worse, make it appear that I was negligent. It was my responsibility to inspect the heat exchanger cleaning and sign off before it was closed, and I was supposed to be notified when to go to the field after the work was complete. I checked the text again and was so grateful to see this was on an old thread with my lead engineer. I suspected this was a mistake but I knew my lead engineer would speak up about this, so I waited for him to respond first.

I waited. . . . Three minutes . . . five minutes . . . *why is he not responding?* I thought for sure he would jump in. I couldn't do this anymore. This was not okay and I was done waiting. I stood up with so much conviction and walked briskly down the hall to the door of my lead engineer's office. "What did you think of that text? That is not okay to say, right?" I asked with an urgency to my voice and fire in my eyes.

He looked up from typing at his computer. "Hmm, what text? I haven't seen any text," he replied as he mindlessly pulled his phone out from his pocket. As he flipped it open and read the thread, I watched his eyes change. "What does he mean they closed the exchanger? Who in the technical group gave permission to do that?"

"No one."

"This is absolutely unacceptable. We have to go down there right now!" My manager grabbed his hard hat, indicating that I should do the same. "I'll drive." Now we were both walking down the rest of the hallway briskly and it felt great to have someone back me up.

That afternoon my lead engineer asked me if other instances like this had ever occurred. I began reviewing to him all the times I had been accused of not proactively monitoring my upcoming reactor catalyst changeouts—which was a false accusation—and, before I even began getting into being left out of communications or accused of not communicating, he took the matter into his own hands. It was reported up the chain and actions were taken. It had helped to have written proof after so many months. My lead gave me permission to review all work items in the morning meetings even though they were supposed to be about updates and not working meetings so everything would be heard in the group and my word would not be questioned again. He also gave me advice I'll always remember as we worked through this situation over the coming weeks together. "Sarah, you don't need to be friends with or have a personal relationship with everyone you work with. You just need to be able to have a professional relationship. Get to where you can have a professional relationship and don't worry about anything else beyond that." This was something I needed to hear for two reasons: it healed the wound from first being told my issue was that I did not have a strong enough relationship with this coworker who was not rooting for me, and as someone who always wants to have a deep connection with those around me, this taught me that it may not be possible in all situations, and I gave myself permission to accept that.

Not long after, a fellow female coworker asked me to come into her office and shut the door. She wanted to ask how I was doing because she had heard about the event that had happened and she had gone through the same thing with my operations lead in her last role. I was grateful she cared about me but surprised to hear she knew about it, since it was all done confidentially. I learned that afternoon that she had reported misconduct and abuse several times in her old role and had never been believed. One of her past supervisors had apologized to her after my situation escalated for not taking action earlier, and since I was the only female working at the control center, she knew it must have been me who had reported it this time. She then surprised me further by apologizing that she had not reached out sooner. She had been watching me and looking for signs to see if I might be experiencing the same but thought I was not and didn't want to taint my perception in case it was only targeted at her and not females. I could tell she felt significant guilt for not speaking to me earlier as she told me about how miserable she had been there and how she begged to be transferred to another control center when no one believed her. I truly felt her heart in her office that day, and was glad to know that the actions that were taken for me also helped her because now she, too, was believed. Together we were happy that any future female engineer would be protected from this particular misery.

A strong shift occurred after this time. I started looking forward to going to work more and I started to let my voice be heard, my udan vayu was expanding.

Twenty-Six

Hurricane Harvey

Driving down the highway I saw an electronic billboard flashing a warning, "A tropical storm is forming in the Gulf, begin to make preparations." I continued on to work and listened as people reacted to the news to determine what level of caution I should take. No one was particularly alarmed—some rain was coming and we needed our hurricane kits ready. The next morning, I opened my door to head to work, and suddenly sheets of rain came pouring down. Afraid that the storm was already here and I would get flooded in at work, I decided I would work remotely. I was notified by my supervisor that this was not allowed; everyone had to report to work, without exception. This was true madness when all our jobs could be done from our computers. A coworker and I decided to call HR, irate that suddenly, the company's policy of "safety above all else," which was preached every minute of every day, had disappeared into the wind caused by the storm. I learned HR really had no power and I was told I could take one of my personal days if I wanted to stay home. It was standard company culture that no one took their personal days, to the point that I had forgotten they existed, so it felt like an odd recommendation. A past version of me might have driven into work, fueled by fear, but now I didn't even question standing my ground. I was willing to take the chance to protect my safety and I was left with an uneasy feeling that my department really didn't have my back. This same day, I had a mini-yoga retreat scheduled for the weekend at Padma's house, more aptly mansion. Since her house was really close to mine, I carried on with these plans and showed up at her beautiful space where I had once signed up for my first teacher training. I needed a retreat after the morning I had just experienced and I was thankful to have a safe space to be during the storm. When I pulled into her driveway that Friday afternoon, the rain had just started up again. What we did not know was that it was not going to stop. This storm would escalate to a hurricane that would forever be known as the once-in-a-thousand-year flood: Hurricane Harvey. By Friday night, it had morphed into a full blown storm. Growing up in New Jersey, I had never experienced so much thunder and lightning in my life. I went to meditate at midnight and the lightning, bold, jagged, slashing through the sky, brought on a mixture of awe and fear. The meditation room was lined with windows and it looked like day, not night. When I closed my eyes all I could see was Mother Nature showing herself in all her glory, and truthfully, I was glad to have a roommate that night. As I curled up in my bed I found comfort in being able to see my fellow yogini's silhouette in the flashing light. It reminded me that we were in this together.

The eight of us on the retreat went to bed like this for four straight nights. By the fifth morning, we were all in disbelief that it could still be raining. How was there any water left on the planet? All we had seen were solid sheaths of rain for days. It would not be until the sixth day that the rain finally subsided and it would take two more days after that before the roads were clear. Our retreat had been substantially lengthened, and I made a mental note to book retreats during hurricane season if I wanted an extended stay. I honestly felt beyond grateful to have been able to ride out the hurricane with this group. We were fed high-quality food the entire time as the couple that was catering the retreat continued to drive in the storm twice a day to cook for us. They had a very tall truck and somehow managed to make it back and forth safely. After the worst of it passed, they said their goodbyes to us, hooked their boat up to their truck and joined the Cajun Navy to rescue people from their homes. My teacher's husband also monitored all of the tornado warnings for us. They were alarming nonstop and I never had to look at a single one. The best part was I had a loving group of people to spend six days with. If I had been at home, I don't even know if I would have had enough food. I would have been alone and probably terrified, wondering if I needed to take shelter from a tornado in my house without a basement. I was no doubt under prepared and kept counting my blessings that I had gotten to spend this time in an elegant mansion instead of alone in a sea of lightning. I was so fortunate to experience this luxury that I almost felt guilty. However, not everyone at the retreat was feeling this way. They had families in the area and they were feeling the need to get back to their home. Most were itching to leave. One person felt a need to go help neighbors, one wanted to see their kid, one needed to help a family member find an open medical facility for dialysis. The list went on. It was through the others at the retreat that I started to understand the impact of what had just happened. We didn't watch the news while there, so I did not yet know the true damage. It would take a full week to process the impact and know how to move forward.

I cautiously began to drive home and just could not believe what I was seeing. Houses just a street away from where we stayed had wet carpets rolled up at the curb, a telltale sign they had flooded and already begun stripping their bottom floor. Tree branches were everywhere, and stop lights were flashing as they were out of service. I pulled into my subdivision, grateful the streets were safe enough to get home. I approached my newly purchased house praying it had not flooded. The anticipation of finding out if the house was okay mounted as I drove closer; I did not have flood insurance. I promised myself repeatedly during the storm that I would get insurance first thing after it passed. As I parked in my detached garage, I felt grateful that at least I still had a dry garage to my name. I slowly walked through my small and overly vegetated porch as my heart beat faster with each step toward the back door. I peeked through the window but couldn't see. With eyes winced, I opened the door and let out a huge sigh of relief. The floor was dry! The house had made it through the storm! Against my own previous judgment, I would never end up calling to get flood insurance as I vehemently promised myself during six agonizing days of not knowing. I ultimately decided if it survived the thousand-year flood, why would I need flood insurance? I called Ryan to let him know the good news: we still had a house and wouldn't have to spend our life savings repairing the bottom floor!

The following weekend was Labor Day and I would be off for this much needed three-day weekend. Ryan and I had planned a grand "honeymoon" in LA—I was looking forward to staying an extra day, soaking up some sun at the beach, our brunch plans . . . it would be my last time seeing Ryan before he left for Japan and we'd wanted to make it an extra-special visit. There was just one slight issue: I couldn't get to the airport and I wondered if the roads would drain by Friday. On Tuesday, all flights were still grounded. I kept anxiously watching airport status updates. On Wednesday, I got an email about my flight. It had been moved up to Thursday. Was I reading that correctly? What? How? Why? This was totally unexpected. The airport was barely open and my flight had been moved up—not back or altogether canceled. I was baffled. It really did not make sense to me then and still does not now. I called Ryan. "Do you think you can take it?" he asked.

"Well our offices are still flooded, so workwise it is not a problem, but I don't know if roads are clear. I am worried I'm going to get stuck on the highway if I hit an underpass that is still flooded." Normally having my flight moved up and offices closed would have been a dream come true, a surprise four-day trip. Yet images of me stranded on the highway kept flashing before my eyes, especially with it being a day earlier. And there was something bigger weighing on my heart too. There were people suffering all around me. The last week had been a whirlwind of finding out whose houses had flooded. The damage was tremendous and I was shocked by how many people I personally knew whose homes had flooded and lost everything. I had invited two families to stay in my guest bedroom. Neither ended up accepting the offer as they had other options, but I really did want to extend a hand where I could. Thousands of families were displaced and at work the situation was also dire. The entire plant had been shut down and it was an all-hands-on-deck situation. I could feel the collective grief. I had never felt such a large mass of people suffering together at once. The closest experience I had to this was 9/11 when I lived in New Jersey, but that was a national grieving which did not have as many direct actions I could take to help. Not to mention I was in the fourth grade. This time I could support, and there was an entire city that needed assistance. It felt cowardly to flee to the beaches of LA and ignore the people in my own neighborhood who had just lost all their possessions and shelter. There was a higher calling for me at this time than seeing Ryan. It was a painful call to make, but I chose not to fly that weekend. We would see each other again. I needed to process what I had just witnessed, and I wanted to volunteer.

Dressers, carpets, books, mattresses, televisions, anything that is in a house was being dumped onto lawns. I was hypnotized by the heaps of endless trash stacked twelve feet high as I drove for miles. It was like every house had been flipped inside out. All you could see were alternating piles of people's ruined things, strapped with warning signs against looting. The environmentalist in me still has a hard time understanding that there was enough landfill space for all the ruined belongings. I felt slightly bothered to see just how much we can accumulate. I volunteered with a group from Rasa Yoga and we joined the forces of people working to carry everything out to the yards; we went to many homes that weekend. It was a mad dash to remove belongings, tear up carpet, cut out the bottom section of sheetrock, and spray everything with bleach before mold could grow. One house we visited seemed to have water damage on the floor and ceiling, giving the impression that everything in the room was wilting. My stomach turned from the smell and I had to take frequent breaks to get fresh air. My heart ached for this family just as much as my stomach. As they ran around frantically lost from the realization that any salvageable items were few and far between, I felt the best thing I could do was stay calm and provide emotional support. This was a low moment in life that no one wants to ever face and I hope that having a group there provided some comfort. I wrongly assumed that this would be the energy of most of the homes we would visit. I've pondered if that is because I would have felt devastation and was projecting or I was accustomed to all the news titles declaring the hurricane a complete devastation. Either way, I would observe that everyone reacts differently and I found myself in the middle of a full spectrum of emotions swirling around me. It was easy to become dizzy and staying steady was more challenging than the physical labor that weekend.

There was one reaction I didn't expect and those who reacted this way typically surprised themselves as well. With all their belongings gone, they were left with a sensation of lightness. I saw this especially with families with a hoarding tendency or who wanted a change but didn't take action. I heard many phrases like, "We always wanted to remodel the kitchen and now we finally will." In retrospect, it makes complete sense. Having the opportunity to start over, or being forced to, can be a wonderful gift after the shock passes. The past is swept away, so old memories and emotional imprints are no longer tugging on our attention with each object we pass, it's another way to leave our material and emotional baggage behind, albeit, a tough one. When the present alone is staring us in the face, the only place to go is forward. I don't know how I would react to this traumatic experience because everyone processes the emotion differently, but I saw that the emotion needed to be processed and this often required support from others. This physical presence of volunteers showing support seemed more powerful than anything that was really done physically. Empathy levels were off the charts as people banded together. They honored others when seeing them at their worst and they trusted everyone would get back up on their feet. I was used to watching hurricanes on the news and listening to all the local heroes. This time the heroes were my friends. These weren't mystical unicorns. The people around me everyday turned into these heroes as we pulled carpet and sprayed bleach. I had friends rescue people in boats. I had friends who consistently delivered diapers and sanitary products to the shelters. I had friends who raised money for families to buy new beds. I had friends who did sheetrocking in homes. I had friends who took in families for months so they didn't have to go to a shelter. The list of heroes was lengthy. There was a true vibe of Houston Strong. The city was embodying the yoga principle of *seva*, selfless service without any expectation of repayment. Seva is considered one of the most important principles to practice for personal development and uplifting the world. I witnessed how this hurricane tore down the town and through seva, uplifted each individual's character. There is a transformative effect for our souls when we give without expectation of being returned a favor. Each time I opened Facebook, I saw another hero emerge. It was so incredible to witness. I wondered what life would look like if we didn't wait for a crisis to extend a hand to our neighbors. It took an entire city to go underwater for me to cancel my flight to Ryan. What if I could be that selfless without people becoming homeless? What if everyone let out their hero more often?

One morning I started scrolling Facebook and a picture of a cat caught my attention. He had enormous eyes and his pupils were extremely dilated with fear. Those eyes pulled on my heart. He was being held up to the camera by a human in an N95 mask and he had his paw which was caked in a thick layer of dirt curled up to his mouth. The caption read, "Lenny the Cat!! This guy!! Needs a home asap!" I had no plans to take in a pet with how much Ryan and I traveled. It didn't seem fair to the animal, but I couldn't stop seeing the unease in those precious eyes. I could probably foster. I sent my friend a message for more details. She is a school teacher and her school had let her know there was a family with three kids with nowhere to go and she had opened her doors to them. They were currently sleeping on cots from the salvation army, and she learned they lost everything. They had a one-story home and they didn't even have house or flood insurance. She went over to help gut their house and discovered they had pets. By the end of the day she had found three dogs, three cats, and three birds. They all needed foster homes for two months until they could get the house back into living condition. I promised to think about it and made sure to call Ryan that night. The next day I opened Facebook and saw another post. It was a video of my friend petting Lenny to show how calm he was. The caption read, "Are you ready for Lenny? He needs a Foster Home ASAP." I read further and saw they would have to bring him to the shelter if no one could foster. I couldn't fathom losing my pet after a storm because there was no one willing to foster for just two months. I wouldn't let that happen to this family, and I wouldn't let this cat go to the shelter. His fearful eyes had captivated my love already. I was not leaving for Japan for two and a half months, so I could lend a hand. I called my friend to tell her I would take Lenny. I showed up that afternoon and Lenny was living in her garage. He was curled up in the corner avoiding all the commotion. He was absolutely stunning.

"There he is!" My friend pointed in the direction of a little ball of fur. "I think he is sad. He hasn't left that corner since he got here. Poor thing even had fleas on him when he was found."

"Fleas?" I repeated. This had not come up in any conversation. I had considered he may pee on my carpets or scratch all my furniture, but I had not thought of this scenario. "Does he still have fleas?"

"I mean he could, I guess," she replied offhandedly. I felt anxiety at the thought of fleas in my home and needing to figure out how to bomb the whole house, with a cat in it nonetheless. I truly did want to care for Lenny but I wasn't mentally prepared for this surprise. Staying true to what I needed, I asked my friend if she could keep Lenny until I found a solution. I could sense her unease as she urgently wanted to get Lenny a better place than the corner of the garage, but she agreed to give me one—at most two—more nights. That night I researched fleas and called anyone who I thought would be knowledgeable. Before long, knowing the urgency I was given, I drove to PetSmart, bought him a flea collar, and went back to put it on him. Then I started calling groomers. Not only did he have fleas, but the fur on his stomach was completely matted together. He had been in flood waters for four days and his long fur did not fare well. Many phone calls later, I finally found a groomer who would not only take a cat but one without proof of shots. I was so grateful. I still am so grateful to that groomer; they had a compassionate heart in the midst of a rare post-hurricane circumstance. The next morning I picked Lenny up and our adventure began. He was in much worse condition than I realized. For starters, about three quarters of his fluffy coat had to be shaved off, he sneezed constantly from a sinus infection, he had lost three pounds (a lot for a cat!), and one of his hind legs was injured. The first four days I had him, he slept in one spot of my living room and didn't move. As I watched his belly go up and down, I thought he was the chillest cat I had ever met, but now I understand he was really suffering and was in a deep process of healing. Day by day his strength grew as did my fondness for him. His personality was pure love. He had a very high trust level for humans and in no time he was curling up beside me. At night he wanted to be in my bed, but his hurt leg and my abnormally tall bed did not make a great combo. Each night he would carefully calculate the jump to the top of Mount Everest and then dig his claws into my comforter as he inevitably slid down the side. This woke me up multiple times a night and left many holes in my bedspread and yet I found the quirk so endearing. He added much needed personality at night.

I received the inevitable phone call earlier than expected. Just one month later I was told the family could take Lenny back. I was so surprised. That was a quick turnaround with how much damage their house had experienced. If flooding was not enough, they unfortunately had also been the victims of looting. I kept recalling what had happened and it just did not add up that they could be ready. I asked my friend, "How did they get the house ready so quickly?"

"Well the sheetrock is cut out now. It is still not filled in and the floors are cement but it is livable," she informed me.

"Do they have beds?"

"No, not yet. They still have the cots."

"How are they actually doing?" I inquired further.

"Things are better than they were, but it is still a difficult situation. I think they don't want to ask you to care for Lenny longer than they have to." There was a sinking feeling in my heart. Did they have the means to buy his food or even their own? My heart was speaking again and this time it told me I had to make sure Lenny was properly cared for. I asked my friend to speak with their family and she graciously sent me the mom's number. I was leaving for Japan soon, so I had a limited amount of time I could foster. While I was pondering this, Lorena walked into my office to chat. She asked what was going on and I told her about Lenny.

"Well, we could keep him while you are in Japan," she replied without hesitation.

My heart leapt at the potential possibility! "Really? You would take him for an entire month?"

"I mean, Daniel loves cats and misses his that he had to leave with his parents when he moved. He would probably love it. If you want to keep Lenny, we will watch him when you are away," she said.

It seemed too good to be true. A solution had immediately appeared. I called Lenny's owner that night. We had a bittersweet conversation where she slowly admitted that they really were not in a position to care for him. They still had a long way to go as a family. She knew it was probably best for him to not come back to the house, but she did not want to put the responsibility on me. At the same time she also absolutely loved him. I let her know I loved Lenny too, and if she would let me, I would keep him. I promised her I would love him every day and give him a wonderful life. Her voice welled up with tears. I could hear how much she treasured Lenny. Between the sniffles I heard her give me permission to care for him. "He is a special cat. You may have already noticed, but he can act very regal. He likes to be the head of the house. His favorite treat is tuna. I poured tuna gravy on top of his food each day." I thanked her for the tips on what he likes and reassured her again that I would make sure he is always cared for. Before we hung up, I asked if she had his proof of shots that I could pick up. "No," she replied. "He has had his shots but the paperwork was in our Bible. All of that was ruined in the flood." I am not sure why cat vaccination records were stored in a Bible, but I like to think it was a symbol of how much they loved Lenny. I cannot fathom how hard it was for her to let him go that day, but I know she gave Lenny a gift. He would have shelter, food, medical care, and love. She also gave me a gift—a priceless gift. Lenny was an angel sent to me during Hurricane Harvey. After two years of living alone, he suddenly gave me a reason to want to go home at night. He was always waiting at the door with a big meow and a welcome head rub. He even looked like an angel. He was a seventeen-pound ball of white, long-haired fluff with a pink nose, ears, and toes. His emerald green eyes shined up at you with unmatched curiosity and compassion. He was kind to everything around him; it did not take long for him to befriend a squirrel on our porch that he spoke to daily, and at night he would get the zoomies as he played tag with the ghosts in our house. And if a cat can be called wise, he was a wise cat. Through watching him, I learned what true acceptance means. He suddenly lost an entire family—five humans, three dogs, two cats, and three birds—had no food through a flood, was displaced from his home, and became physically ill, yet he accepted all of it. He rolled with the punches and adjusted quickly to his new home. Watching him gave me my greatest lesson in contentment. He showed me what contentment in action truly looks like as he purred through each day. The flood gave me a priceless gift. I gained a companion and Zen master in my house.

Ryan would meet our new family member Lenny after his time in Japan, seven months after I adopted him.

Twenty-Seven

Papa

My phone lit up on my desk; my mom was calling me at 1:00 p.m. A shiver shot up my spine. I instantly felt something was wrong. I planted my feet, took a breath, and answered.

"Hi, Sarah, honey. Are you sitting down?"

I reached behind me with my free hand to find the chair's armrest and carefully lowered myself down until I knew I was squarely in my seat.

"I am sorry to have to tell you this at work but um, um Papa passed away this morning." The shiver in my spine strengthened. *How could my grandfather be gone?* Tears effortlessly rolled from my eyes. Time had stopped—yet it hadn't. My brain filled with fog.

I couldn't stay at work. I shot my supervisor a text explaining that I was headed home, and I didn't know when I would be back to work. I grabbed my bag and swiftly walked to my car as tears streamed down my face as I drove home. I passed an operator while I was crying and thought he must be judging me for overreacting about work and I didn't even care. When I walked into my house, I saw the picture of my papa in our family photo. *How could he be gone? Was it real?* It was so unexpected. He went to the gym that morning as he always did. *How could this be?* It wasn't a situation where I could say he was in good health. After developing scarlet fever from strep throat and being bedridden for the entirety of second grade, he had always had a precarious heart condition. Yet he had never let this get in his way. He had a deep passion for life and was the most active person I knew. With the exception of watching him take a handful of pills each morning, I never linked the words *Papa* and *sick* together in my mind. No one who knew Papa ever considered him sick, and as we watched him overcome every symptom he faced, he seemed invincible. The shock of the news really came from seeing that although he had surpassed every statistic, he couldn't be invincible forever. I wanted to talk to Ryan, I checked the clock, it was only 2:00 a.m. in Japan—surely he was asleep. I texted him with a message to call me in the morning, before he went to work.

After what felt like days, Ryan finally texted. He was up! I called immediately and I know he was already shocked by my short response time and that I was calling instead of texting. It was unfortunate to have to tell him right before he went to work across the world, but death does not wait. I was fully prepared to tell him that he did not have to fly home for the funeral. I let him know that no one in my family expected him to make the trip, but if he wanted to, my parents were willing to pay for the flight. I could hear sorrow in his voice as he spoke. He didn't waiver for a second. He was coming home. He wanted to be there for me. And more than anything, he loved Papa as his own grandpa. He had actually lived with my grandparents while on one of his internships in college and he became the grandson they never had. During this internship, I learned that my grandma was making his lunches every morning, Papa and him were watching all the college basketball games together at night, and Ryan was preparing everyone dinner. He was acting as their personal chef. I was now the second favorite grandchild which was good with me. Ryan could have his glory and they could have their grandson. I knew they had enough love for both of us. Needless to say, Ryan was almost insistent that he was coming home. There was no indecision in his mind. Only one option.

My dad started booking flights. It so happened that my mom was in Ireland for a business trip, my dad was in New Jersey, I was in Houston, Ryan was in Japan, and we all needed to get to Ohio. Papa brought my family back together in a major way that weekend. His love was the center point that united us.

Stepping into my extended home once I landed was a powerful moment in my life. It felt strange to not be coupled with a holiday or summer childhood trip. In the center of the kitchen table were twelve beautiful red roses and tied to a kitchen chair were five large colorful balloons. Papa had celebrated a birthday and wedding anniversary the previous week. Still in shock, I felt like an outside observer to the scene. How many people are as lucky as my grandma to say they received twelve red roses for fifty-six years on their anniversary? How many seventy-seven-year-old people are as lucky as my grandpa was to say they still receive balloons for their birthday? My grandparents never took a year for granted. They always celebrated life. They taught me the importance of a year in so many ways through their relationship. They believed it mattered to acknowledge every milestone that passed in its entirety.

Ryan arrived home the next day. He was so loopy from lack of sleep that he kept repeating himself and his words weren't stringing together coherent sentences. No one had the heart to tell him he wasn't making any sense. We were all just so glad he was there. I couldn't believe he was in front of me in the flesh. I was not expecting to see him for three months and yet here he was. An unexplainable joy washed over me, and temporarily numbed my sadness. Was I allowed to feel this happy when my papa had just passed? I was once again experiencing simultaneous joy and sadness. They ebbed and flowed through me with intensity as I processed this moment. Over the last few months, I had come to understand that two different things can be true. Life is a paradox. I felt somewhat guilty being reunited with my love when my Grandma was grieving hers yet I knew she would want me to be happy. She and my papa were also high school sweethearts and they'd always had a soft spot for that similarity with Ryan and me. I knew she wanted me to have fifty-six or more incredible years with my love too. I was with Ryan and it was okay to feel happy as well as sad this weekend. *Papa had given me a true gift. He did always know how to honor life.*

I was as proud of my papa as I was heartbroken at his funeral. So many people showed up that the funeral home could not find enough chairs. It was standing room only. People of all ages, social classes, and backgrounds came. The most striking part was that nearly no one referred to him by name. Everyone used the same familial language. "Your grandfather was like a dad to me" . . . "like a brother to me" . . . "like an uncle to me." My mom was his only child and I was his only grandchild, yet there was a room full of "extended" family. One moment I will always particularly cherish is when a young girl my grandparents were tutoring passed us in the receiving line.

Her face was really sullen until she looked up and saw me. "Oh, I have seen your picture on the wall in their house!" she exclaimed.

"Yes, that is me. I have also seen your picture on their refrigerator."

She looked starstruck and confused as she processed this information. I do not think it ever occurred to her that I had heard of her too. It clicked that we had a connection. I could see in her eyes that his passing weighed heavily on her. It was irrelevant whether our relationship was friend or family. It was irrelevant how long we had known him. We had both been touched by Papa's love.

He left a heartfelt legacy. He had sincerely cared about everyone who crossed his path. He was in no way gone. He still very much lived in me. He lived in everyone who came to pay their respects. He once again taught me that life is to be lived. Life is to be celebrated.

Ryan flew home the next day. It was a fast turnaround, but I was filled with gratitude that I got to see him at all. I was left contemplating what my legacy was going to be. How was I going to be? Ryan and I may be physically separated, but how was I going to celebrate this next year of my life? Was it a coincidence that Papa passed in January, the month of New Year's intentions?

The year of Sarah had turned into the years of Sarah, and it was time to honor the precious gift of the next year ahead with some momentous intentions.

Twenty-Eight
Hiroshima

While we were in Japan with my parents during Ryan's internship, we visited Hiroshima to see the Peace Memorial Park that commemorates the atomic bombing of the city. On the ferry ride there, I wondered how the Japanese feel that Americans now come as tourists to see the horrific suffering our country once created. I feared we would not be welcomed as I am still scarred from the time an English waiter at a pub in London gave my family a difficult time about the Boston Tea Party. As our ferry approached, our first sighting from across the water was the Atomic Bomb Dome. Only the dome part of the building was intact above some half-standing large cement walls, which still give the impression that this was once an architectural marvel. Because it's right along the water's edge, it's prominently visible; the city chose to never repair it to serve as a reminder for how the entire city was once in ruins. Amid the newly constructed surroundings, it is an impactful entrance to the city that leads to introspection before even stepping to shore. Its decimated aesthetic added to my apprehension of us visiting. When we met up with our tour guide once on land, we found she was so incredibly sweet. She was absolutely thrilled that we had come to see their city and I let out a small sigh of relief. We began to walk along the streets to the memorial, and a Japanese man passing on a bicycle greeted us. "Hello! Where are you visiting from?" he asked.

"America," we responded. I held my breath.

"America! How great. Welcome! Welcome!" he cheered as he rode by.

I let out a full sigh, feeling relief that we were indeed welcome, and was ready to see the city. Our first stop was the museum, and as we entered, we came to a large stone next to the doors engraved with this passage:

> War is the work of man.
> War is the destruction of human life.
> War is death.
> To remember the past is to commit oneself to the future.
> To remember Hiroshima is to abhor nuclear war.
> To remember Hiroshima is to commit oneself to peace.

—His Holiness Pope John Paul II

I was so moved by these words. *Yes, we must commit ourselves to peace*, I thought. This was the same message that ran through yogic texts. This message became even more evident as we moved through the museum and observed a preserved outfit covered in blood stains and a tricycle that was carrying a three-year-old toddler. Between all these objects were videos playing with interviews of survivors describing the aftermath and what life was like in the first weeks after the destruction. It was a museum that brought us to tears and reached out to my soul. It required us to see human suffering. It also taught human resilience. The most incredible parts were the displays that showed how the citizens reacted after the bombing. It was incredible to see how they bonded together to heal the sick. The ways in which they dealt with their grief. After the situation started to stabilize, the city focused on rebuilding. Through a timelapse video which showed Hiroshima's reconstruction, we learned that the city was remade with incredible speed, and underlying all of this, it was rebuilt with a strong desire to start fresh. The citizens accepted that they had a part to play in why the bombing occurred. They took responsibility, forgave those that caused the suffering, and got back on their feet. The city wanted to learn and never repeat the past. I now understood why we were so welcomed as Americans and was impressed by their ability to accept their part and forgive another country.

As part of the intention to never repeat the past, the last part of the museum showed current events and how Japan supports efforts to eliminate nuclear warfare. I noticed a framed display with a picture of President Obama and a paper crane in this room. Our tour guide came over to me elated. "I see you noticed the picture of President Obama. We really like him here. He was the first sitting US president to come visit Hiroshima. Many people thought it was very honorable that he visited. It was a real sign of progress," she informed me. I was happy to hear that but surprised he was the first.

Later that same day, the 45th US president tweeted: "North Korean Leader Kim Jong Un just stated that the 'Nuclear Button is on his desk at all times.' Will someone from his depleted and food starved regime please inform him that I too have a Nuclear Button, but it is a much bigger & more powerful one than his, and my Button works!" I would have always been deeply distraught to see this type of language from a world leader, but it seemed that much worse while we were viewing the horrid aftermath that occurs from an atomic bomb. I felt embarrassed that this was the leader of our country. We were standing in a city committed to peace while our president was joking about this extremely serious topic. Having power over a weapon that can kill hundreds of thousands of people in seconds and wreak havoc on lives for generations to come is not a game. It made me wonder if we had made any progress. What would it take to truly evolve? Our tour guide asked us what we thought of the tweet. She was genuinely curious with an open mind. As I sat back and observed my family discussing this tweet with our tour guide, I felt a glimpse of hope that maybe we have made some progress if we're able to have this conversation. Not enough, but some nonetheless.

Our day in Hiroshima is one I will forever treasure with its overwhelming tone of peace in the air. I have never felt anything else like it. It cannot be explained; it is something that has to be experienced. The people who live there seem to have a deep sense of forgiveness. They understand the importance and they understand true resilience at a cellular level. It reinforced for me that on my healing journey, I want to stand for peace. I was comforted that I was on the right path with my yoga training because the world needs more people who are not divided from themselves . . . so we don't divide from others. I felt a renewed vision to dive into what peace can mean on a much deeper level and on a larger scale. In the museum gift shop, I bought a bell with a handle that is Sadako Sasaki holding up a crane. She is one of the most famous child survivors of the bombing and is known for folding over one thousand paper cranes. Now, these origami cranes are a symbol of peace. I wanted this bell as a symbol to remind me to expand my perspective around my problems. I hoped it would remind me to forgive myself for a decision that led Ryan and I to living apart. I hoped it would remind me to consider all the ways in which I need to forgive myself. I hoped it would remind me to reflect on where I need to forgive others. It was clear to me that I needed to first find peace with my own situation, if I ever hoped to see world peace. I hoped it would remind me to keep training in yoga to find more ease and share this with others.

How could I bring more peace into my life and therefore the world? How can I commit to peace?

I still take a moment each morning to acknowledge this bell during my morning meditation. I gaze at it with deep gratitude for the life I am privileged to live. My passion for yoga resparks and I remember that I am learning to become peace.

Twenty-Nine

Guilty

One day when my mom was visiting Houston she asked me the standard questions of how work was going and had we heard when Ryan would graduate. I provided my consistent answer that was honest—work was fine, my new role was better than my last one, and I just hoped I was really making a difference for the environment. To make a positive difference in sustainability is always what I wanted from day one but knowing whether you are creating a shift is often convoluted. As for Ryan's graduation date, we still didn't know when that would be yet he thought he could graduate a year early. He had strived for this for some time but a PhD is really up to the timing of research results and the professor at the end of the day, which means it's a black hole. I did mention that I had let go of my aspirations to move to Los Angeles. As much as I had dreamed, it no longer made sense especially with a potential internship Ryan would have in DC. Our circumstances were very different than a few years prior, and I had to admit staying in Houston was for the best.

"Yeah, that makes sense. I am sorry this has turned out to be longer than you wanted. You know sometimes I feel guilty . . . I feel responsible," she said from a soft heartspace. I could tell that she had been holding onto this thought for a long time.

"Yeah, I know," I said after a short pause. The rest of what I should say escaped me.

"I do not know if I told you the right things in the beginning. I was trying to help you financially and to have all the facts to decide, but I often feel like I might have done the wrong thing by telling you that. Maybe you would have been happier in California," she added.

I really felt my mom's heart in this moment and it was meaningful to me that she was willing to share how she'd been feeling. I'd suspected she felt this way and understood why she might. I could hear that in a genuine way she was acknowledging that there was validity in the path I had wanted to take to follow my heart. This was a powerful acknowledgment yet underneath the surface of how everything looked, I knew how everything unfolded was not her fault. She did advise me to the best of her ability with what was known at the moment. I empathized with what she shared and tried my best to reassure her that she could forgive herself because this wasn't on her. I felt I should have had a longer response, but I was lost for more words. I could feel her pain and I was dealing with mine too, but I did know our separation was not my mom's fault for telling us that Houston was financially better. That was true. It would have originally been much easier to process emotionally if there was someone to blame. The truth is we had to make a decision when there were still unknowns, and no one could predict the future. Ryan and I could have made many more choices after that decision to live in the same state too, but it always turned out to be more complicated. Life involved more factors in it than simply being together. We were no longer innocent fifteen-year-olds with plenty of time to chase each other in the school soccer fields until we collapsed on our backs to be mesmerized with the shapes of clouds. We had our eyes set on many new adventures and we had to learn along the way. Through my yoga training, I had learned that to get to a state of empowerment, I must take full responsibility for all my decisions and life circumstances. I was the reason I was in this situation and I was not a victim of anything. My heart spoke to me very clearly that California was calling, but I was too afraid to listen. I was the one who silenced my inner guide. I had to take responsibility and forgive myself that fear led me to make a different decision. I was also fully responsible for making any future decisions for where I would go next.

I was ready to let go of the victim mentality and take responsibility for my world. For without this, there can be no hope of healing.

Thirty

Follow

After Ryan graduated, we both knew we would likely move to where he found a meaningful job and that was likely neither in Houston nor Los Angeles. It just made sense. I was not working my dream job and I had always felt like an outcast around Houston. Yet, my mind kept telling me I should not be following Ryan's career. My thoughts would run through my well-established programming. *Is following your husband being a strong woman? Can I still consider myself a feminist? Why don't I know where I want my career to go, then I could lead if I did? Am I compromising by finding another job to be together?* I had been raised to be a strong, intelligent, and self-sufficient woman and I was feeling like I might be in conflict with this image. These thoughts started when I began searching for jobs in Los Angeles. As Ryan's graduation approached, the self-sabotaging thoughts began growing stronger. I waited for them to subside, which they didn't. In a vulnerable moment, I revealed my inner dialogue to Padma. She seemed far less concerned about these thoughts than I was anticipating. I honestly thought she was going to say, "Of course you should be driving your own life. You should get clear on what you want and then move toward that." I was waiting to be told I was wrong. Instead, she paused and looked at me with soft, loving eyes and asked, "Well, what are you trying to follow? Are you following your heart?" This question threw me off. What was I trying to follow? My heart or my mind? I had been thinking so much about following another career that I was at a loss on how to answer this. Padma could tell I was fumbling and continued on. "I mean, are you following your heart because you want to be with Ryan, the person you love dearly? Is that what you want for your life? . . . All that really matters is that you are following your heart." It took some time for the lesson to sink in for me. Day after day, and week after week, I asked myself the questions Padma had posed to me. Understanding what I was following required a complete perspective shift. I was focused on the wrong priorities when thinking about leading and following. The external job or form of what it looked like was not key—was I following my heart, my inner compass?

The answer, of course, was yes, I was following my heart. I could let go of my self-judgment that I did not know where I wanted to steer my career or that I had not found a job that called to me so I could direct where we would move. Because the deep truth was that I did know. I could hear my heart whisper that it did not want my career to move up the corporate ladder. I'm sure it wanted to speak louder but I was only allowing a whisper to arise as I was not yet ready to own this story even though it had been true for a long time. Every time I searched for jobs, I saw again that I did not want to live learning how to be more assertive in a conference room and proving my prowess each day at a computer from 9:00 a.m.–5:00 p.m. (and let's be honest, this looks more like 7:00 a.m.–6:00 p.m. or worse the higher you climb). I wanted to open my own business. I had always wanted to, and instead of the restaurant I dreamed of as a little girl, now I wanted to open a yoga studio.

In the deepest part of my being, I knew that I could accomplish my dream from any location.

All I needed to do was follow my heart, learn to let it speak, and eventually allow it to shout.

Thirty-One

Life is Short

I had often heard "life is short" from adults as I was growing up. We each have our finite number of breaths and heartbeats that will make up our life. Each moment is precious and we get to choose how we will show up. The wise elders then warn us that life goes by in a blink of an eye. We are each presented with the question: How will you spend these sacred seconds?

When doubt would creep into my psyche about our long-distance relationship, I would sometimes wonder if life was too short to live this way. I would start to wonder if we should prioritize being in the same zip code. One day I asked Ryan, "If one of us died tomorrow unexpectedly, would you regret our decision to be long distance? Do you ever worry that you would have regrets?"

"No, I would not have regrets. We made this decision because it was the best thing for both of us, and we made the decision together," he answered without skipping a beat. I could hear the confidence in his voice, but I questioned if he would have regrets again.

"Are you sure? You really wouldn't second guess our choice?"

He, again, explained without wavering that we had considered a lot of factors when we made the choice and there was no reason to look back. I respected and envied his confidence. One of his biggest strengths is being able to listen to his inner voice, make a decision, and not spend an ounce more energy on the choice afterwards. His steadfastness brought me comfort. I was glad he would be at ease if anything happened. What he had was complete acceptance. This was a state I was struggling to fully achieve. I logically accepted our situation and could reason why it was beneficial. I even had felt full acceptance regarding our situation recently, but it would inevitably waiver again. As I teetered back and forth, I knew we had both been given a chance to work on our passions so that we could move closer to mastery. I also knew from the last few years that being in the physical vicinity of any individual did not equate to living a richer life. My emotional body on the other hand was still not 100 percent on board. I was still, after all this time, subtly grasping for what could have been. That is not true love. When true love is present, there is nothing that you feel the need to change. All is already perfect with all its imperfections. I wanted to drop the resistance in an instant, but it was taking quite some time. It felt like I just could not completely surrender.

There was a little more to unbury to meet freedom. I would dig deeper.

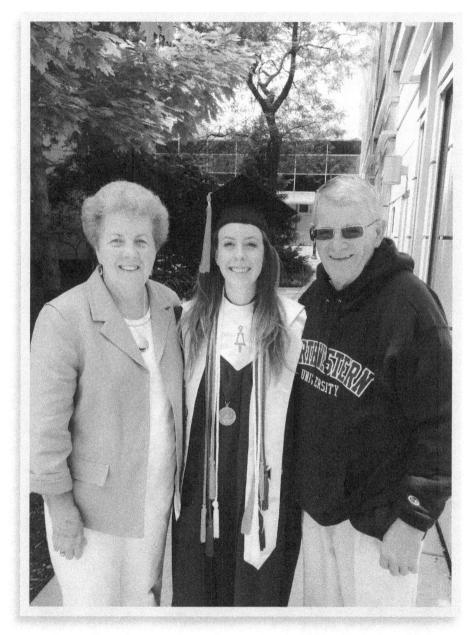

Papa, Grandma, and me at my college graduation. As a high school teacher and first-grade teacher, respectively, they were always teaching me lessons and were overjoyed to celebrate this milestone with me!

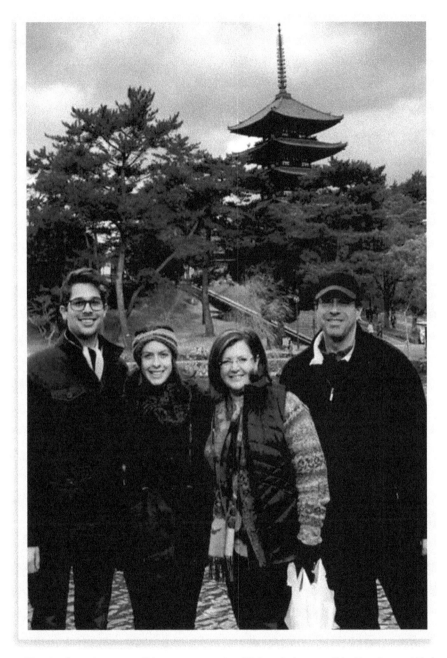

Exploring Japan with my parents. This picture with the beautiful Pagoda was taken in Nara on New Year's Day.

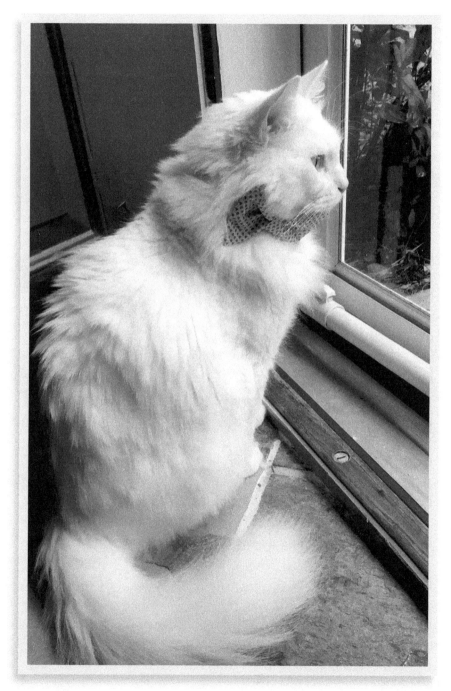

Our precious and majestic Lenny who was such a gift.

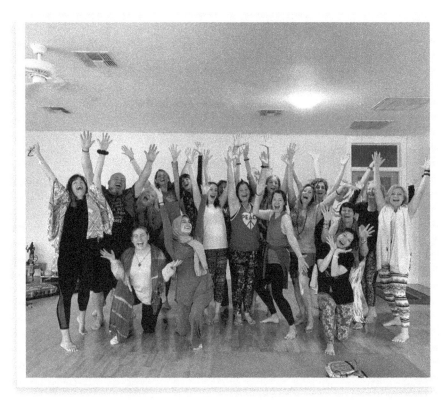

The Rasa Yoga community who I dearly miss seeing every day.

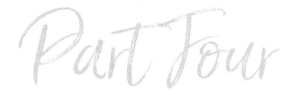

Healed

Non-attachment and love are one and the same

—SWAMI RAMA

My best friend pointed across the playground to a boy. "Sarah . . . Sarah, look over there, but don't be obvious! That's Ryan; that's the boy I have a crush on." This was fourth-grade recess so I was not exactly scouting for boys or putting a lot of weight into my friend's words. I looked over just to be a good friend and was quite surprised by my reaction. My immediate thought was *Wow, I wish I had seen him first and could have a crush on him.* Rule number one of fourth grade: You can't have a crush on the same person as your best friend. Energy radiated from him and the sun hit his skin in a way that created a golden glow. His hair was spiked with gel and frosted tips. Believe it or not, this was the cool style at the time. I felt a sense of awe, a pure connection. My younger self could not understand why I felt this way, so I didn't try to understand it. Anyway, he was too popular and my friend already had a crush on him, so I didn't think any more about it as I rushed over to hop on the swings.

It would be years before this memory resurfaced and I would remember that initial encapsulating feeling of time stopping when I looked at Ryan. It wouldn't be until high school that his radiant energy would once again catch my eye.

Thirty-Two

Four Days

I was perfectly happy, scooping equal amounts of rice from the rice cooker into five individual tupperware containers while Ryan finished stirring the curry across the island from me. I expected to smell the earthy tones of the curry but it was the aroma of his roommate roasting chicken in his beloved cast iron skillet, lovingly nicknamed Casty, that kept wafting my way. We were all packed into the kitchen of his tiny apartment; the classic white walls, milk-colored floor tiles, and non-descript countertops boasted a subtle, off-white hue, reflecting years of use by college students. The near perfect LA weather breezed into the kitchen through the open window. I sighed as I realized this would be what Sunday nights would always feel like if I lived here full time. Even as I shoveled five lunches worth of curry into only five plastic lunch containers, I decided to let myself pretend this was my life.

This was what our honeymoon weekends had started to evolve into since I had made the executive decision that all of our trips needed to be at least four days long. The decision was not a sweet couples discussion focused on coming up with a compromise; I had forced my voice out and declared that this was a must. I had gained enough experience to know that two days was too short, and I had gained enough courage to ask for what I needed. Ryan figured out how to make this happen for me with his responsibilities and so I had to do the same. Although my job was now more flexible due to decisions I had made over the previous years, it was uncommon to work remotely and asking for this flexibility was quite bold for the time. The company had certainly progressed on their employee accommodation practices since I had started, but the vibe in my office still reverberated the message "you are only working if I see you working." Luckily, after several meetings, I was granted this extra time in Los Angeles every other month, and I did not concern myself with how it would reflect on my reputation or take the chance for granted. Looking back, I just wish I had asked sooner. I was concerned about asking for too much because I felt like I was always making requests. I had asked for a month of unpaid leave to go to Japan, to be on the Northwestern recruiting team, to create an employee-based sustainability group, and to attend a Dale Carnegie training, just to name a few. I had been granted everything I had asked for, and I didn't want to push my limits. In retrospect, I can see clearly what is true; the worst thing they could have said was no. If there is one thing I really learned during this time, it's that one has to ask for what one wants. No one has time to let fear limit them. No one can read our minds and opportunities are not normally (if ever) extended to us on a platter. Ask. Ask. Ask. The worst case scenario is the situation remains the same.

Our extended trips notably enhanced my overall happiness. Everything was easier, especially adjusting to the time zone. Although our visits could still feel like minihoneymoons, our days of being tourists were long gone. We had transitioned seamlessly to slipping into each other's lives, sometimes picking out the best produce at the local grocery store or joining friends for brunch and sipping taro boba tea afterwards. By now, we knew each other's friends and they knew us. I often went to Ryan's climbing gym pretending I was a regular and he came to my yoga studio where everyone felt like they knew him. When Ryan visited me, I had a list of house items that I needed help with. The time we gained was exactly what I needed to start to navigate our world with acceptance.

One month Ryan and I could not make the four-day trip work. We both had obligations that made it necessary to see each other just on the weekend. Then we added salt to the wound when we found a great flight deal for early Sunday and booked it greedily, making our trip even shorter. When that week rolled around, I was angry that I had booked a flight that essentially left us one day to see each other. I promised myself I would never trade time for money again. It just wasn't worth it. I felt so sad that we would have such a short visit when we had been thriving with the longer stays. My entire body felt heavy from going against my own advice and decision to move away from these fleeting trips.

The Friday morning before this one-day trip, I was dragging around the office dejectedly when a new department head was announced for my group. This wasn't particularly unusual. Most roles at that level rotated about every two to three years in the company. What was unusual was that to introduce himself, he scheduled a one-on-one meeting with me. As I walked into his office, I was reminded of past meetings with previous managers as I saw the same corner office I had been in before with its big glass windows facing the plant and large V-shaped mahogany desk with the laptop facing away from the door for privacy. But his office chair was out of place—instead of behind his desk which is customary, he had parked it in front of his desk. He had put us on the same side;

the large, black leather seat was intentionally placed so we could talk without the large desk between us in an open gesture which gave me a lot more confidence to speak when he politely asked about my life outside of work, if I was willing to share. Bringing up my situation was always awkward, but for the first time I decided to be upfront. When he found out I was in a long-distance relationship, he reacted much differently than all my previous leaders. Instead of commenting on how hard that must be or praising me for my strength, he asked what the company was doing for me. He wanted to know if they had worked with me to make this doable. Had they discussed how to use the flexible hours policy with me? Was I allowed to work remotely? How frequently had managers checked in to see if I was supported? I was truly surprised by this change of pace and it was a relief. I caught him up to speed that I had recently asked to work remotely two days a week every other month. He was glad I was allowed to do that, but he felt they were not doing enough—especially when I told him it had been ongoing for four years. He had been long distance from his family once, had experienced the agony, and understood the importance of being able to visit with quality time. Because my job could be done completely remotely, he said I should go to Los Angeles and work from there for a full week. Before I left, he again made sure it was clear that I should work with my supervisor to find a full week to go visit and then we could work on how frequently I could do this afterwards.

I thanked him for his support. As I walked away, I thought about how I really wanted to say, "I need that week this week. Can I change my flight for this weekend so that I can work remotely?" I was not brave enough to jump on his request so fast. It did not seem professional when he had just been so caring, and it certainly wouldn't have been viewed as professional to mention that I was really missing my husband at that particular moment. I did however realize that although I had asked for something I needed, I might not have been asking for enough.

When I thought I might be asking for too much, there was space to dream bigger. I could have been asking for full weeks. Although my stay this weekend would not be extended, I left filled with more hope than before. There would be a week in the near future that I would go visit him. It meant a tremendous amount to me that a leader had finally offered a solution to help make the long distance situation easier. He will never know how much it meant to be told I could be flexible with what location I work from and not have to initiate the request myself. I did not mind asking, but I felt much more seen when management took a proactive approach on behalf of the company. It provided an unexpected sense of relief. He was a strong example of a caring and effective leader.

As we bridged the miles, time together remained a precious scarcity, a reminder to always ask for what I truly needed, so that one trip I would stand at the kitchen island sealing ten tupperwares for our week.

Thirty-Three

Flow

We were wrapping up the final topics in my last meeting of the day and I was psychically sending everyone the message to not ask questions—which is only polite etiquette on a Friday afternoon. Miraculously the meeting finished on time as if the Universe was on my side, and I walked straight to my office, snatched up my keys and lunch bag, and slipped out the back stairwell to ensure I didn't run into anyone who may have remembered they had a question. As I turned on the ignition, I looked up to check the time on the dashboard and was relieved that I would be right on time for my yoga workshop. I briskly walked into Rasa Yoga, taking in the calming aroma and the stark contrast of its slower-paced atmosphere compared to work. With two minutes to spare, I quickly slipped off my work onesie (the plant-issued FRC coveralls) revealing my yoga outfit underneath. My friend next to me looked over in confused awe, "Did you wear your clothes underneath all that? Now, that's next level!" Yes, it was. It had only taken me three years to get to this workshop on time—the same workshop I had walked out on, head hung in shame from complete failure and exhaustion. I finally had found my flow, the mysterious flow state that is mentioned in yoga studies that encompasses the sweet spot between boredom and fear. I no longer felt like I was living two lives with yoga and work. I had molded the life I desired. Everything was integrated. Yoga was work and work was yoga practice. They were like my breath.

Inhale: Receive a new work assignment.

Exhale: Take a yoga class.

Inhale: Present a proposal.

Exhale: Meditate.

Inhale: Silently name my breath at a meeting.

Exhale: Create a PowerPoint diagram for a yoga workshop.

It was this seamless flow that ultimately enabled me to approach my next big opportunity.

I was sitting in our regular Monday-night yoga-psychology lecture when Padma announced that she would be hosting her first three-week yoga intensive in Austin, Texas. "It's going to be a total transformation for anyone who attends. You will not come back as the same person." My eyes might have actually widened as I absorbed her announcement. It sounded absolutely incredible to leave life for three weeks to reflect, reset, and revitalize. Even as I sat there, I could envision myself journaling next to a peacock, every afternoon, after a morning of asana and meditation practice. I immediately wanted to be there but I was dismayed; how could I go? I only had three weeks of vacation a year and I had already signed up for a three-week trip to India. I couldn't fathom a way but I had learned over these last few years that if I opened myself to the possibility, clarity might just reveal herself, so I decided to keep an open mind and heart. Months passed—I continued to keep an open heart—yet I continually felt a heaviness every time the retreat was mentioned. I envied my friends who were retired or had created such stability in their careers that they could effortlessly leave for a month. It was unreasonable to compare myself to friends with twenty-to-thirty-years more life experience than me, so I allowed them to become beacons of hope that this level of flexibility was achievable. I desperately wanted to be there with them and challenge myself to this three-week transformation. My desire was growing and each time I felt my heart contract from a frustrating thought I caught myself, put my hand over my heart, reminding myself to breathe, and allow trust and an open mindset to soften my heart. I would wait to be guided through the closed door I was pining for.

It was just two months before the date approached when I suddenly gained a higher perspective, like viewing a treasure map, I glimpsed where the key to this door might be hidden. At the time, I was responsible for leading a month-long audit, and I was told that I would be given a new role in the company shortly after. My work responsibilities seemed to be lining up to where I would transition jobs right around the timing of the retreat. I realized that if I gave my company enough notice, the timing was promising to where they could plan my job transition around this vacation. The only barrier that remained was my lack of vacation days. I knew I would have serious regrets if I did not try to attend, so I made a firm decision that I would ask my supervisor if I could attend using my yearly training days. I even announced it to a few friends to keep myself accountable. I had to try. I had to ask. After all, I had learned the lesson that I must ask and the worst thing they could say is no. If they said yes, I could go on a trip of a lifetime.

This was my most daring ask yet. It was one thing to ask to visit Japan for a month because your husband is working there. It was entirely another to ask a Fortune 10 engineering corporation to go on a three-week yoga intensive by yourself as your yearly training. The oddity of this was compounded by the fact that I did not live with my husband. I'm sure it confused my management that I would spend so many vacation days on a trip where I would not see him. I even baffled myself, but I had to follow my heart. I wanted to learn how to be fully present, a masterful yoga therapist, and a retreat leader myself someday. This trip was at the center of my dreams and therefore worth pursuing fervently.

I was so nervous when I sat down in front of my supervisor, an agenda of every day of the retreat accounted for and informational flyers pressed tightly into my sweating hands. I even had testimonials from yogis with impressive job titles—a brilliant suggestion from Padma when I discussed this with her.

Surprisingly, my supervisor received the information really well; I could thank my excessive preparation for that. I was ecstatic and although my mind told me not to get too hopeful because the final approval was several layers above him, I somehow knew in my gut that I was going. We waited to hear from the higher-ups and three weeks later my initial proposal was denied. But my supervisor really was invested in supporting me despite being perplexed as to why I would possibly desire to go train with no cell phone and laptop connection to the outside world. We collaborated and brainstormed different ideas we bounced over to management, all receiving rejections. And then, one day he came to my office with the announcement I had been visualizing: "You are approved to go." I was absolutely thrilled! I trusted I was in a flow state, and now knew I could hold the vision, as I saw myself going on that trip. Maybe we wore them down, maybe they felt too much time had gone into the decision to abort, or maybe they truly saw the value, but it was ultimately approved without the details figured out. Gratitude oozed from me!

Mixed in with my intense gratitude was nervous energy. I wanted to go, but questioned whether I was prepared for this experience. It was called an intensive instead of a retreat because it was designed to shine light on all the places we are attached to in life. It was not designed to be a relaxed, restorative yoga retreat. The days began at 5:00 a.m. and ended at 9:00 p.m. Daily practices would include no contact with the outside world, days of fasting, periods of time in silence, no sugar, caffeine, alcohol, or meat (luckily as a vegetarian, that one was easy for me), and certainly, no snacks (that one was hard for me). The time was designed to draw our attention inward as opposed to grasping at the outside world. The goal was to work through the obstacles in our lives that were preventing us from living fully present and free. I wanted to live in the present, but I really was not sure if I had the mental discipline and capability to surrender my sleep schedule, diet, and routine to this practice for three full weeks. What I did know, is that I was willing to try.

During a meditation before the break of dawn, I sat up on my zafu (meditation pillow), hugging a yoga shawl around my shoulders, shielding me from the morning chill. We were all sitting in rows, candles casting the only light in the room, silently repeating our personal mantras to ourselves, when I miraculously realized I was alert. Finally, my head wasn't bobbing up and down from falling asleep between instructions. This was in stark contrast to the retreat two years prior, where I had never acclimated to rising early. I was pleasantly surprised to find I was able to participate with relative ease. I was riding my wave of immense gratitude which allowed me to surrender to the moment and enjoy the full experience; challenging sleep schedule and all. I was even grateful when my tummy rumbled with hunger in bed after two days of fasting. It was miraculous that I had manifested official approval.

During this retreat I could see how far I had come from the Sarah that had attended the retreat two years prior. It was clear that my training had paid off. I felt more grounded, I had more clarity around what it was I truly wanted, and finally, my nervous system was calm. This was a pivotal moment for me; I reflected back on where I had started, full of anxiety, and could see my progress. I could see the results were evident in my life. I no longer struggled to make the early-morning yoga workshops. I could communicate more assertively and set needed boundaries when working on my projects or with managers. My back was healed and I was pain free. I was teaching yoga regularly and had even taught my first yoga workshop. I had once worried that I could not complete my two-hundred-hour teacher training before I moved due to the obstacles of being in a long-distance relationship. Now I had completed that, two Ayurveda certifications (a sister science to yoga), and was halfway through my five-hundred-hour training. I rarely take enough time to celebrate my successes and my strength tends to be seeing where I want to improve. However, during this time, I did take pause to see myself. It was almost impossible not to, with the stark contrast staring me in the face. Past Sarah probably could not have dreamed that this transformation could take place in two years. It was important that I could be proud of myself. After all, yoga is about cultivating self-love. For we cannot love others if we do not first love ourselves.

What I had the chance to see during these weeks of retreat, was that I had created a life I loved. Two years ago, I was not only struggling through a retreat but I was applying for jobs in Los Angeles, in order to run away from my misery. I knew when Ryan graduated that it would now be hard to move because I had cultivated meaningful relationships, a great environment, and a supportive routine for myself. But I knew it wouldn't stop me either. I was not attached, and would hold the flow state to wherever life brought me, but I would deeply feel the loss of what I loved.

In the end, I received compensation days for the overtime I worked during the audit, along with a holiday, ensuring all my time was accounted for and paid. By opening my mind to seemingly impossible logistics and asking without hesitation, the locked door finally opened. And I saw that it had been open all along.

Thirty-Four

Dockweiler

The wind blew through my favorite sundress along with the top layer of beach sand, leaving the rest for me to squish between my bare toes. Sunglasses couldn't block out the perfect warmth of the sun beaming down on my skin. We were at Dockweiler State Beach with Ryan's main friend group. The plan was to have a beach day filled with frisbee throwing, swimming, and eating—and then we would end with a bonfire. I was immersed, for that moment, in the type of weekend I had always wanted, frolicking the beaches with Ryan and friends. The frisbee was flying between people running every which way. The competitive spirit amongst the group became even more evident as we watched a low flying plane overhead. "Watch me!" one of the guys shouted out. "I bet I can hit that plane with the frisbee!" We collectively laughed—there was no way he could throw that far. "That's like me saying I could throw this frisbee all the way across the beach to the Chevron plant!" Another friend mockingly shouted back.

My body froze at that word: Chevron. Of course, I had forgotten how close we were and that the refinery was only five minutes from the airport. I looked up over the sand dunes and noticed sections of tanks visible from where I was standing between foliage. They were painted tan to camouflage with the landscape as part of their initiative to not be seen, heard, or smelled by the community which was highly emphasized in my interview with them. I was transported back years to when I stood on the other side of the fence line, amongst the tanks, during my interview, watching the employees ride their bikes around the refinery, my guide pointing out the silhouette of the beach in the distance. Personal time travel is real and I was back in time before I made the phone call to them saying no. A silent pain tore through my body at the thought of how often I may have stood here on the beach had I made a different decision. To think about how the trajectory of my life would have gone was overwhelming because nothing would have been the same. Two lives splintered in opposite directions the only solace being that perhaps another Sarah is living the second in a parallel universe. But I was here, this Sarah, standing on the warm shifting sand, taking in the foundation I had created for myself going too far down the lane of *what could have been.*

I had traveled down the road of what-ifs enough by now and I had learned too much to let myself go down the road of grief again, over one word that represented what could have been. I inhaled the salt-infused air and forced myself back to the present, the place that was bringing me so much joy. I reminded myself of all the incredible memories I had made over the last few years, that didn't include the other path. What had been—had been. The past was in the past and it was a magnificent past that also included sporadic beach days. Today the gift was to enjoy the beach day of my dreams, knowing that tomorrow would bring its own mysteries and wonders.

This, I learned, is the way of healing. There is no finite place of *healed*. It is a winding road where one word can slingshot us backwards into our wounds. Yet progress can be easily identified by how quickly one can recover; how quickly I could return to myself in the present moment with mercy, forgiveness, and compassion.

Thirty-Five

On Call

One afternoon my supervisor came to my office. He was fiddling with a rolled-up piece of paper in his hands. I wasn't sure if he was going to use the paper or if it was soothing his nerves to have something to hold, but I found it curious how he moved the tubelike structure every time he talked. He informed me that a new position had come available, but it was a completely different position than the one we had been discussing for the last nine months. This one was for a pipeline coordinator. I immediately tensed up, knowing this role was typically a position that required being on call. In our conversations together, I had made two requests that were requirements of my next job. The first one was that I didn't want to be on call, and the second, was to be by a major airport. These were the same requests I had required before my current role to improve long-distance logistics. Many of my peers warned me that making these requests was career suicide, but it had worked out great for me so far. This time, I had also casually mentioned that I thought I'd enjoy working in supply chain. My supervisor justified that the department thought I should really consider pipeline coordinator because it was in supply chain (punctuated by a heavy reminder that

I had asked for this), had great visibility, and would challenge me to build new professional skills. The only drawback . . . it was on call. He had checked the extent of the on-call obligations, and assured me that I should only expect two to three calls a week, after hours. He needed to know by the next day if I would be open to this role or still wanted to wait for the analyst position.

I put all my energy into maintaining a straight face, but given how my closest friends have often told me, I have no poker face. I wouldn't have been surprised if my inner world was written all over my outer expression. My thoughts were running wild. *Why so quickly?! Why was I just hearing about this now? We had been discussing this for months and this never surfaced.* I felt like I was facing an ultimatum and my heart was starting to race.

A good friend of mine happened to be in the role at the time. I wasted no time in texting him to ask how he liked the position. He answered right away and I could hear his distinct British accent and dry humor as I read the text. "Oh boy, Sarah," he replied. "I can't get out of it fast enough. It is a hell of a job. I get so many calls at all hours of the day. Not the best job if you want to have a life."

"They are considering me for the position," I replied.

The mood completely changed. "Oh, well it is not that bad. We have just had a streak of bad luck lately and I was exaggerating—no you'll be fine. You will learn a significant amount in it and it is a very respected position. You will also be responsible for marine movements which is a skill you do not get to learn in many roles. Let's grab lunch and talk about it." His answer had a strange mix of honesty and desperation for him to get out of this role as fast as possible, and I was his ticket out.

I then walked directly to my work wife Lorena to gain her insight. "That is definitely not a Sarah job. Do they know you? It is nonstop calls. The most of any coordinator! I do not know anyone who has not gotten burnt out in that role. Definitely not a great work life balance." My heart rate was starting to beat faster. My flow was slipping away. How much I had learned to integrate work and yoga was about to be tested.

I went home that night to reflect. All of the emotions from my first year of being on call had erupted from the depths of my being like a geyser. My memories insisted that I not go back. I had set a boundary that had greatly helped me and there was no need to reopen that door. The one issue was that rising to the highest version of myself is always a priority for me. The more I reflected, the more I could see that the analyst role that had been discussed for nearly a year, was not going to bring me any new skills or growth. It would barely be a challenge for me. The on-call role was going to skyrocket me into another realm. It was going to require extensive customer interfacing, learning supply chain, navigating ship movements, coordination among ten different companies, and managing my work life balance to name just a few. Plus, it was in the back of my mind that having the word supply chain in the title would make it easier for me to get a job in another company later on since this was a universally recognized field. By this time, the possibility of transitioning to another company was heavily on my mind.

My whole body was trembling as tears pooled in my eyes. Was I really going to choose to be on call? Again? After all the excruciating pain it brought the first time? Past emotional patterns were tugging at me hard. I could feel them—*big time*—but I knew what was best for my self-transformation. I was able to face them and say: It is okay. I got this. I promise. I am going to take the on-call role.

I had decided. Period.

Immediately after, two poems surfaced in my mind. I do not write poetry so this was not a familiar occurrence for me, but they just came through—without any paper or pen. The words were so clear and strong. They kept running through me as if providing me a message. I listened to them as I stepped into the shower before bed. I let the words continue to repeat in my mind as I rinsed off the past determined for a fresh beginning. When I got out of the shower, I effortlessly wrote the poems down on paper not forgetting a single word when often I cannot remember what I just said I need to buy at the grocery store.

Samsara

You held me with your powerful grace
So swiftly you saved me

I was nearly broken, torn to shreds
And lost beyond what one can see

I prayed that night with all my might
to express my sincere thank you

Yet here I stand once again at the door
of lessons which I still need

I feel the all too familiar space
and what you are requesting of me

You've struck a chord deep in my core
My mind screams no and my heart beats to the haunted score

But I will listen and try again to return your gracious gift
And hope that this time I find my own way out free

Obstacles

I saw the darkness
I saw the tunnel
I saw the swirling plight

I knew that this was a life choice point

I wanted smallness
I wanted comfort

but I chose to serve you right

I stood upright on that dark night
I walked straight into that tunnel
knowing on the other side would be light

The poems provided me with undeniable comfort and affirmation, that although this would be hard, I had made the correct choice *for me*. When I got out of the shower, I reread "Obstacles," and caught my breath when I realized the words that flowed out of me could also be describing death. A deep understanding dawned on me in that moment. There *had* been a death; I was ready to surrender a part of my ego that I no longer needed. The inner work I had completed rendered me a new person; and this person did not need the layer of protection that separated me from the demanding on-call roles. It was time to relinquish a boundary that had, at one time, served me by benefiting my health and happiness. I had grown so much, that boundary had turned into a box that was now limiting my potential. It was time to step back into the fire and release that pattern of fear from my consciousness. As I reread the words once again, I could see clearly how this decision would sustain my work and yoga balance—because I was *living* yoga.

There was no looking back. No regrets. I had made my decision. I was clear that no matter what happened, I would fully accept my decision because it had come from my heart. It was this unwavering acceptance that led me to contentment when the job proved to be as challenging as my friends had described.

In the end, I excelled at this role. I was determined to master the art of being on call while integrating my yoga, work, and travel life. The decision to take the harder path would prove to pay back dividends over time.

I dove into any remaining darkness in this corner of my humanity and I gained a new sense of freedom.

Thirty-Six

Reunited and Alone

My coworker leaned into my office doorway all bug-eyed, "Hey, did you see the first few cases of the coronavirus have made it to America?" At this point, everyone was still calling it coronavirus and I don't think COVID-19 as a name had even been publicly shared yet.

"I heard that might be the case, but I haven't looked into it," I replied nonchalantly, going back to my computer screen.

"Yeah, I've been watching the Johns Hopkins map. It's really neat what they put together."

I looked up quizzically, revealing that I had no idea what he was referring to. "You haven't seen it yet?!" he exclaimed. "Oh, you have to see it." Over my shoulder, he gave me precise instructions on how to pull up the website, introducing me to the interactive Johns Hopkins map which showed the relative amount of COVID-19 cases around the world with different-sized circles over the various regions. I just wish then that I had known this would be one of the last times I'd ever have a coworker interrupt my work day or stand beside me to chat. I could have savored the moment more.

I scanned my screen noticing large, overlapping circles all around Asia, and just a few tiny dots in America. Over the next few weeks, I repeatedly pulled up this map, checking it like I did the weather app right before my wedding day. I was in shock and awe at how rapidly the virus was spreading. I watched as Italy and then Seattle's circles started to resemble those in Asia. Even as Seattle's outbreak grew out of control, I did not understand that my life, and everyone else's, were about to change forever.

As chaos ensued, reality struck with the notion that traveling might not be safe. This did not fare well for a long-distance relationship, and it certainly started to weigh on me that there could be several months that Ryan and I would be separated. I could only describe my relentless feeling tone as an endless sigh, and I was consoled by my own random assumption that this would be three months tops. But those Johns Hopkins map circles started growing at rapid speed to where one afternoon Ryan called to tell me UCLA was shutting down for an indefinite amount of time. He couldn't work anymore so he was flying to me the next morning because he didn't want to risk airports shutting down. My mood transformed in an instant! My joy was overshadowed quickly by concern that an entire university had just been shut down. But picturing being locked down, just the two of us, won out, and my giddiness returned.

Ryan made it to my front door two days before the state of California went into full lockdown. He was finally with me! Our lives had collapsed into the space of our house over night and time had frozen while the world spun frantically around us. It was a powerful experience of the principle that everything is temporary. The good, the bad, and the ugly will all change. We had been apart for so long that it had become hard to fathom that it would actually end and here we were with four years of time to catch up on, and we had every minute of every day to do so because of lockdowns. I was struck with the realization that truly anything can happen in life and there is only the present moment. As strange as it all was, it was honestly magical. Oftentimes I felt guilty being happy when there was so much fear and loss occurring with the virus, but being reunited with Ryan was the best gift at that moment. Our lives had simplified drastically with a level of free time I had never experienced. Ryan made us homemade meals every day, and I started eating better than ever. I even started an at home workout three times a week and actually lost the five pounds I had worked a decade to lose. It just went to show that if I want different results, I have to take different actions.

Our typical marathon packed evenings were now free to do what we chose —albeit limited to the confines of our home. Our favorite pastime became Tuesday movie nights. While I didn't actually own a TV, we improvised, propping my laptop on a side table by our couch in our living room which had the perfect evening ambiance. Every Tuesday night, I would eagerly tear open the piping hot kettle corn bag and dump it into our largest bowl as we hopped onto the couch, Lenny curled up on the floor below us. With some imagination, we pretended we were at the movie theater, and it felt so rebellious to indulge like this—on a Tuesday. I was so completely unused to the concept of open evenings, that I felt a mixture of freedom and discomfort simultaneously. It was a potent time where I learned that it was okay to not have to do, create, or produce; I could let myself be; and being with Ryan, after all the days we had been apart, was the cherry on top.

Ryan placed an epic grilled cheese down on the table for me one evening, a true favorite of mine. The toast was perfectly browned and crisp with cheese melted to oozing out the sides of the bread. I picked it up, ready to experience that first incredible bite, and as I crunched into it, my bliss was interrupted by a buzz from my work phone. I ignored it, taking another bite, needing to use my fingers to separate the cheese from my mouth as it stretched from the toasted bread. It buzzed again and again and again. Texts began rolling in like I had just announced I was selling tickets to spend a day with Taylor Swift. I sighed as I slapped my sandwich down on the plate. I just wanted to savor my dinner in peace while it was still grilled to that crunchy perfection. I gazed over at my phone that had practically moved an inch from its spot on the table from all the buzzing. I knew I had to look, and in my heart, I knew all the messages were going to be related to COVID. It was too good to be true that my role had not been impacted by it yet. Everything was temporary and my simple life was over.

The emergency work meetings began effective immediately. With the shutdowns and everyone working remotely or not at all, this meant our demand for chemicals that made tires went to zero overnight. No one was driving. No one was buying. We had millions of pounds of chemicals flowing in and nothing flowing out of the pipeline. Our tanks filled up quickly. We scrambled to get more barges, but every one was purchased (we were not the only ones in this situation). We got to the point where we sold ships and barges for free—FREE! And that still was not enough. Storage became such an issue that oil prices went negative for the first time in history. This became one of the few headlines that was sensational enough to be heard among the mounting daily COVID case count and how Tom Hanks and his wife were doing after their COVID diagnoses in Australia. I was now working around the clock and with Ryan home, he unfortunately also woke up every time my phone rang in the middle of the night. I was fortunate that

Ryan brought me homemade matcha lattes during meetings and helped make sure my limited free moments were full of laughs to create some distance from the situation.

This was a unique time period in our lives. I would have never guessed there would be a time that I would work from home and Ryan would be there without needing to work. It lasted a solid two months and we soaked up every minute of the simultaneous worldly craziness and household stillness until change was inevitable, once again. A loyal universal truth we can always count on. The day came that Ryan was informed UCLA was planning to reopen the labs. I was not eager for him to go back, and I did not respond to it with giddiness. I was resistant and wanted our intimate COVID reunion to last, and there were plenty of excuses I could draw on to validate my wish. UCLA's plan was not official, and I felt there was a risk he could fly back to LA and they wouldn't actually reopen. We also did not know what the true risk was for him to fly in a pandemic, which brought on a lot of fear. Now we know flying was one of the safer activities people could do with the ventilation, but that was not known yet. Ryan reminded me, once again, as he had every weekend we had flown home over the years that he had to get back to graduate so we could be together permanently. He reminded me that he worked so many hours so that we could be reunited. I eventually (very slowly) got on board and accepted that he had to return. Selfishly, I didn't want our ideal COVID reunion bubble to burst. I knew when he left, that I would be facing this new COVID world alone.

The months after Ryan left were like none I had ever experienced before. I went from working at a campus with six-thousand employees and going home to a yoga community of thirty close-knit people to seeing almost no one. Speaking to employees at grocery stores became a real event. In just a few months, that transformed from a typical side conversation to potentially my only face-to-face interaction with another human in a given day. This was a strange world. Whereas previously, in our long-distance relationship, I had felt lonely, now I felt alone.

My office opened fairly early in May 2020, just two months after lockdowns, so I was going into the office about twice a week—but I still did not see people. Walking down the hallways felt like it was perpetually 7:00 p.m. because I never saw a soul. We rotated who went in each day and all meetings remained virtual. As for my yoga studio, they also started to open. The class spaces were limited and they had implemented about every COVID sanitizing protocol known to man. There was only one protocol I couldn't reconcile which was that you were to wear your mask to your mat and then you could take it off. By this time, we had learned that the main way COVID was transmitted was through the air, so I felt taking our masks off for an hour was not going to stop the spread. To further paint a picture of where this was in time, Houston's hospitals were over their capacity and vaccines were months away. I faced an ethical dilemma. Should I return to the community, connect with people, and get out of the house for sanity, or stay home in order to help limit the spread of the virus? It was a hard choice to make with the enormous isolation I felt, but I stayed home. I felt it was my responsibility to help limit the spread while hospitals did not have enough beds and ventilators. I was fortunate that I was able to take the classes virtually, but it was not even *remotely* the same. And not teaching my own class pained me the most. My yoga community meant everything to me and having differing opinions from them was painful. I was called to use the voice I had learned to strengthen over the last few years and go against the grain. This tension that led to separation stung sharply but I did stick to what I felt called to do in the moment.

Ryan had returned home many times before, yet this time my loneliness was not simply fueled by my yearning for us to not be long distance. I felt so much more. I felt loneliness on a global scale which was beyond us. I wished for him to be there because I missed everyone. Instead of a resistance to our reality, my viewpoint was more of being awestruck. Where I would have previously felt like a victim, I saw where this was more of a personal choice. I really felt empathy for everyone who lived through the pandemic in relative isolation. I have always been pretty good at being alone as a highly introverted, only child. I love sitting by my cat reading a good book with a hot cup of tea. I'm renewed by quiet, alone time, but this was next level. Months on end for reflection became daunting, even for me, who was deeply acquainted with myself. While I was grieving the loss of laughing with friends at the yoga studio, I was really getting the best yoga practice there is: Could I really be by myself? Some yoga lineages will say that when you never feel alone, that is when you know you are really connected and enlightened. For when we can tear down the hard exterior shells we create for protection, we find the entire universe is in our heart. We are a microcosm of the macrocosm. This is true evolution to be able to find everything from within and not grasp externally. It can also take a lot of practice to feel this infinite space within us. Before these months, I thought I was rather good at loving being by myself, but the duration really illuminated to me how much more I can practice being at peace. This was not one quiet evening or a designated period of days for a yoga retreat. This was an indefinite amount of time where the ending was uncertain. It was difficult—truly difficult. The days required connecting to my inner source of joy. In previous years, I learned how to stand without Ryan by my side. Now, I was learning how to stand without anyone by my side.

Although it hurt, and I don't recommend practicing this unnecessarily as we are meant to be social, I am grateful to have seen clearly where I still had work to do, to see all the places where I relied on others for happiness, and to see where I had room for more self-love.

For ultimately, we do not take anyone with us in the end. We are all born and die alone. And I wished for my alone to be filled with more happiness. Complete and utter bliss.

Thirty-Seven

Dreams

Ryan always shared my passion to think beyond the now and try to live out our deepest desires in order to ultimately leave the world a better place; so much better that it was beyond what we could imagine achieving. In Sanskrit, this intention or resolve is called *Sankalpa*: a vow to live out one's heartfelt desires. We were strong at supporting each other's Sankalpas, which is why we stayed long distance for so many years. We agreed we didn't want to get thirty years down the road having lived a life that was built on a foundation of heavy regret.

One afternoon, while sorting through the Houston guest room closet—which had become our de facto storage space—I realized we could leave behind some excess belongings and lighten our load for the move to our next home. Surrounded by stacks of boxes I had not touched for years, I felt confident there was something to donate after all this time. Of course that only happens if one doesn't open the boxes.

Peeking into the first box, I picked up a large blue binder laying on top. Flipping it open I realized it was a record of a high school scholarship I had received which contained all of my academic and athletic achievements. I flipped through the laminated memories and paused to read my college admission essay. The words struck me harder than I expected, so I read them again. I sniffed, wiping away a tear. *Why am I getting so emotional reading this essay?* I felt silly sitting here in the guestroom, rifling through my childhood memories, and crying. Then it dawned on me—I was living the vision that I had written about nearly a decade ago. I was in the midst of the reality I had said I wanted when I had so often wondered how I ended up in this position. The words popped off the page as the last sentence read, "My dream is that during my lifetime 'a world in which machinery chugs on, day and night without stop, making Gluppity-Glupp' will only be a fictional story for children to read about a time long ago when nobody cared but the Lorax." The writing prompt was to describe a fictional character that inspired me. I had always loved *The Lorax* by Dr. Seuss and was devastated, as a child, when the last Truffula tree was chopped down. This became a full-circle moment for me as I read the next line of my essay. "When I realized the magnitude of this daunting task, I recalled a verse from *The Lorax*, 'UNLESS someone like you cares a whole awful lot, nothing is going to get better. It's not.'" It sunk in for me how true these words were, as the magnitude of the dream I held was daunting and expansive. No wonder these years had brought forward challenges! No wonder I was working in manufacturing for one of, if not the, largest fossil fuel companies in the world. And what's more, I realized with blinding clarity—I *did* care. And my work enabled me to help others speak out about what they cared about too.

It took an old essay to remind me of something very important: I had chosen this. I had never envisioned living out my purpose would involve living apart from Ryan or working for an oil and gas company but this life, the way I was living it right now, was part of what I created. Dreams are tricky like that. When I envision my dreams, I'm always feeling triumphant inside at how that peak moment will feel; absolutely glorious! Yet the journey to the dream's peak moment is really where the action lies and the journey doesn't always feel warm and fuzzy because it requires me to step out of my comfort zone, or more often *zones*. I realized when a dream made me shake and quiver in fear it can be so easy to forget I am in the middle of realizing my desire. As I sorted through what to keep and what to donate, I reflected on whether it was possible to reach a revolutionary dream, without facing one's demons. Perhaps it is in facing our demons that allows the peak moments to be so gratifying? As I packed my essay safely back into its box and then found a place high on a shelf for safe keeping, I wondered: *Can you really have a high without a low?*

I could feel in my heart that I did still care about creating a more sustainable world—watching the last Truffula tree fall to the ground with that telling "Whack!" still devastated me. I loved our world and wanted to see an evolution in sustainability. I was grateful for the experience I had in manufacturing plants to see the complexity of the systems that source our luxurious lifestyles, yet I was ready for a new path because through my yoga training I had grown to see sustainability from a new angle. Manufacturing, pollution, and overconsumption of resources is a symptom of a larger issue, not a cause. It had become clear to me that when one is content inside, there is no longer a need or even a want to grasp and possess so much externally. I had come to understand that the solution started with each individual person. To really see a sustainable world, I had to first ask myself if I was using my energy and the resources I was privileged with, sustainably. I needed to work on my own inner peace before changing the world.

Padma would always say that the most important question to ask ourselves when approached with any decision, whether it was to eat another chocolate bar, train for a marathon, or switch careers, was "Is this sustainable?" When I sat with this question, along with the memories of days gone by, on the floor of my closet, I knew that my current role as pipeline coordinator was not sustainable for me. I felt like a lone salmon swimming upstream in a river meant for trout. It was draining my energy and my inner voice was telling me that it was not my ultimate calling. I could not continue on the path I was leading and be my highest and happiest self. I wanted to design a more sustainable life for myself and then inspire others to design this for themselves. The time had come to start manifesting a yoga school. While I knew it would be perceived as a complete pivot, I also knew at the core of both my engineering days and yoga life, my passion would always be to see a world where we master how to use our energy sustainably so we could make the world a better place.

For this new dream, I made a decision: I'd make sure not to forget where I was headed, despite the twists and turns. I would let my intention, my Sankalpa, carry me through the obstacles that would inevitably lead me to self-doubt before reaching a new level of freedom on the other side. My Sankalpa would be my inner guiding light when I inevitably would have to face feeling internal discomfort in order to grow.

I was comforted by the steadfast reality that Ryan would be my other guiding light, cheering me on as he always had to ensure we didn't stray from the path towards our dreams.

Thirty-Eight

Bliss

Over time, I had settled on a nighttime routine that served me well. After my last emails were sent, and I checked the front and back door to make sure they were locked, I would go into my bedroom, turn on my Himalayan salt lamp as well as some of my favorite yoga music, then lie on my back, on the floor, which allowed Lenny to curl up around my head, and read. This was such a peaceful time of my day; the salt lamp emanated the perfect soft, pink hue across my room as I read, accompanied by the purrs of Lenny, draining all anxiety and tension left over from the day.

This was *my* time, and it was sacred.

One evening I turned on my music and, before I made my way to my back on the floor, I found my body involuntarily swaying to the music. Lauren Daigle's song "You Say" came on, and I felt an immense amount of joy arising from within me; I let the music take me wherever it wanted to go as I wound down from my long day. There was no explanation for it—but there was a tingling all throughout my body, *This is pure bliss!*

I was elated and that tingling turned into a state where I felt like I could suddenly do anything! Out of nowhere, I was overcome with a spontaneous desire to do a forward flip! I knew I could do it, even though I hadn't done a forward flip in years—or maybe never? But this joy was so strong so I felt certain I could land a forward flip! I placed one foot in front of the other, ran halfway through the room, planted my hands down on the floor as I kicked my feet into the air like I was seven years old! In mid-air my logical mind kicked back in, bringing a healthy dose of adult terror with it.

What are you doing?! My brain shouted at me.

You can't do this! You're going to hurt yourself! This room is too small for flips! I came tumbling down to the floor as my mind questioned my ability, causing me to disconnect from this unexplainable burst of blissful energy. As I lay there on the floor, I laughed out loud. What had possessed me to actually want to run around my house doing flips with such freedom and self-abandon? How had I for a moment fully felt beyond human limitation?

I recalled the man at the gazebo and his message to sing and dance. Then I remembered the bhakti yogis, whirling dervishes, and wise beings who had spoken of the power of dance and music. I felt this must be the experience they were trying to share in their teachings. *This is what it feels like to feel completely content, to feel whole.* A smile spread across my face as the realization warmed my heart. The song that was playing may have helped me make this internal shift but I knew this wasn't caused by just a song. This was the result of my yoga practice and being able to be fully aligned when the moment fell into place. Somehow, I had connected to my true inner self where there was freedom to experience infinite joy caused by nothing outside of myself. As I made my way back to my corner of the floor to take up my book and snuggle with Lenny, I realized I had reached a new level of understanding in my being. To those who have never felt this sensation before, I probably sound crazy. But for those who have, it's likely agreed that this is what happens when we allow ourselves to connect to the wholeness that is inside each and every one of us.

I wish I could say I feel this infinite well of love all the time but it comes and goes. I've listened to "You Say" so many times since and although it holds a special place in my heart, I've never gotten the urge to try a running forward flip again! I do, however, feel grateful knowing this love and invincibility will return in other ways, and it is always there and available to me, even when I lose my way. I'm grateful I put in the time to align with myself enough to where I could feel it rise up.

That night I felt it. Pure love. Pure Bliss. Connection to my soul.

Thirty-Nine

Virginia

Humid heat engulfed me as I stepped out of my car and grabbed my face mask to shop at Rooms To Go. Thirty salesmen in matching uniforms faced me outside the door in a perfect U-shape—it reminded me of the ballerinas in *Snow White* waiting for the prima donna ballerina to take front stage. When I realized the prima donna was me, the potential customer, I was tempted to run back to my car and wait to be recast as a stagehand. Because of the pandemic, I had barely seen a living soul in months, let alone been in the company of full staff. One of the supporting salesmen practically leaped over to me, starving for a sale, and once we were safely socially distanced inside, I felt slightly more at ease—but only slightly. Masked and eight feet away, I was able to relax enough to listen as he listed off all my options for couches, and for the first time in five years, it felt real that Ryan and I were going to live together again. His graduation date had moved around so much, especially when UCLA shut down for COVID, that we didn't know what to expect. But the day had finally come, and we had an official end date. He had accepted an offer to work for the US Naval Research Laboratory based in Washington, DC, out of graduate school, and together we made the decision that we would move to Virginia. For the first time, I was following my heart.

While he was finishing up his PhD, I asked my company to work remotely for one year and they graciously granted this request. I had prepped to request this for quite some time, considering how I would phrase my request and prove I could deliver on my commitments, but COVID-19 made the approval process much faster, as I had already proven I could get the job done working from home. It was no longer a revolutionary request with the state of the world, but having chosen to take the pipeline coordinator role was still beneficial. That particular role had three offices pre-pandemic, so managers were already calibrated to not seeing the employee in that role everyday. And post-pandemic, what was the difference between working from a home in Texas or one in Virginia? The pandemic seriously uprooted everyone's life, but I feel very grateful that it benefited Ryan and me in many ways. We were able to spend a few months together in Houston before he graduated, and it provided the opportunity for us to move to Virginia together and keep my job. This meant we could explore our new town together which was ideal. I was so relieved that I would not be living alone in lockdown or in a long-distance relationship for much longer. I was so grateful and I never lost sight of that. This was the beginning of the end of many phases for us, and I empathized, more than ever, for all the people feeling lonely at that moment. I knew what it was like to feel lonely, and I knew how jubilant I was that my reign of living alone was nearly complete. My heart went out to everyone still living in the mystery of when they'd be able to leave their houses. It really was the uncertainty of everything that caused so much of the angst. And although COVID was not over, I was finally given a date to mark off on the calendar as to when Ryan and I would share a home.

The day I was scheduled to fly to Virginia was finally here! I stepped out the door with my oversized backpack strapped to my back, pulling two large suitcases, and our gigantic cat Lenny in his travel carrier. For the first time in my life, it had been months since I'd been on a plane. It was a strange feeling. The price of my plane ticket proved that I was not the only one who hadn't been traveling much. Lenny's ticket was ridiculously priced, costing more than mine, since pet fares are a flat rate that don't swing with supply and demand. Preparing Lenny for the flight could be a book, in itself. I had fixed up our house to sell, found a friend to drive my car occasionally, left keys with our realtor to watch the house, sold furniture in Texas, bought furniture for Virginia, and said my goodbyes with ease, but coordinating how to fly with a cat had been tedious and nerve-wracking. Cats are notorious for being stressed by change, and this proved true for Lenny as well. Getting him to take medicine was near impossible, plus, he was seventeen pounds which puts him at the perfect weight to barely fit into any carrier that suitably fit under a plane seat. My saving grace was that the middle seats were being left empty because of COVID, which provided me a little leniency with my gentle giant poking out from under the seat. Through the process, my mind kept telling me I might not be able to travel with him alone. Could I take him out of the carrier through security and get him back in his carrier? I could barely get him into the carrier at home where things were calm and familiar. The treat bribe no longer worked—he was too smart. I had recurring nightmares of him jumping out of my hands and sprinting down the terminal for the nearest hiding place. *If only Ryan and I could fly together, then this would be easier.*

It had been five years. Five years of managing everything on my own, and doing quite well, thank you very much! But here I was, my mind still trying to convince me I needed someone else, trying to persuade me that I wanted or even needed a safety net. Yet I noticed one major thing that was different. I was acutely aware of these thoughts. I saw the thoughts that were pulling at my mind and I knew, deep down, that I could do this alone. I did not resist. I faced the obstacle before me. I took it one step at a time by planning well ahead of the flight.

I was happily surprised that Lenny had slipped right into his carrier like a slinky that morning. The immense preparation and incessant pleas directed at our vet for other ideas on how to administer medicine had clearly worked. As I stood there on my front porch, with a few suitcases of my essential belongings and Lenny, I looked around our yard, and studied its abundance of trees, honoring our time together, in case I never came back home. A pandemic had taught me that anything could happen and I'm glad I said my goodbyes, because I never did return. I clicked our gate shut, signaling the end of an era that had begun five Septembers ago. I was leaving Houston a significantly different person than when I had arrived.

My best friend from Rasa Yoga was waiting in the driveway. I climbed into her car, put Lenny's carrier between my feet, and strapped myself in for the ride, not knowing what was ahead. It truly meant everything to me that she drove us to the airport. I wouldn't have wanted it any other way. She had been a pivotal part of my Houston journey and her love was sending me off to my next chapter. I wanted to extend her a hug so much yet we followed safe COVID protocols. It was such a strange time to be leaving so many people who I had come to admire and not be able to give hugs or in many cases even see them in person before departing. The transition felt much like ripping a bandage off; in no way gentle, but very real. It was actually happening.

Lenny successfully meowed, vocalizing his discontent, for the entire plane ride. He stopped as soon as we landed. Since everyone was afraid of each other, I didn't feel the need to engage in apologies for the excessive meowing. When Ryan met us at baggage claim, it was all so surreal. I had to continually remind myself that this was not a weekend destination trip—we landed at our new home where we were going to be together without an expiration date. He picked us up in his new car he had bought the week before and my mind could not process that this was not a rental for vacation. This was really our car, and we were headed to our next place to live.

For so long, it had been "someday" or "when" and someday had finally come! The weather was nearly perfect. A seventy-degree, sunny fall sky with no clouds. Despite this, I was shivering on the drive. Having come from over one-hundred-degree weather in Houston, this felt like winter. The thick skin I had grown in Chicago during college was far gone and my body and mind were trying to recalibrate to this transition. Everything felt new, but the trees alongside the road brought some nostalgia. After ten years, we were back on the east coast, and I recognized the familiar foliage alongside winding roads. It resembled where we grew up in New Jersey, and it surprised me. I was ecstatic to see more greenery, hiking trails, and people moving at a faster pace. We smiled and shared stories as we drove past the trees to the apartment.

Sometimes, in life, we are fortunate to experience moments of perfect contentment, or in the yogic tradition, *santosha*. Life felt complete to me on that car ride; there was no need for any more dreams or ambitions because we had arrived. I snapped a photo of us all together to capture the present moment of wholeness. I was still beaming as I stepped through the door of our new apartment; white walls, white carpet, a fresh start. I was so elated to be there. I had to keep remembering it was real.

On the way home from the airport I had seen a sign that welcomed me to Virginia. I chuckled when I saw the state slogan that said, "Virginia is for Lovers." I looked at Ryan lovingly and whispered a prayer of gratitude.

It sure was.

We were in the right place.

Forty

What if?

I used to feel angry that Ryan had the chance to live on the sunny coast of Los Angeles but I didn't. When we moved, I truly felt left behind. I couldn't see that this story wasn't true, and that I wasn't left behind. I had trouble reconciling what had happened. Why did it have to happen? Was there another way? Then one day I contemplated a question I had been offered in yoga training, "What if everything that happens is for me?" What if Ryan and me having to move to different states was for me all along?

So, what if all of this had happened for me? Relaxing into the luxury of looking back, I could see how much it had benefited me. There were so many gems that emerged because we chose to follow this path. I had gained confidence to stand by my own decisions. I had grown to find a deeper sense of self-love. I had created a wonderful life for myself and maneuvered adult challenges like buying a house on my own. I couldn't even imagine what life would look like had we stayed together because it was such a large fork in the road, but I know there were positive things that might not have occurred. Would I have followed my dream of becoming a certified yoga instructor as quickly if we had been together?

What if I had never met my yoga guru because I went to California? What if I had never found the peace and contentment I gained from training at Rasa Yoga? Where would Lenny have gone after the storm? Would Ryan have been able to immerse himself as much in research if I had been waiting at home every night? Would we have gotten a month to explore Japan? Could we have afforded to buy a house in Virginia? Would we have taken for granted being under the same roof? Would we value each other having our own hobbies and experiences to the same degree? Would I have learned the skills to choose happiness?

The answers to these questions were simply hypothetical, yet they brought me an appreciation for what unfolded.

What if life has my back? What if we can trust that every moment is exactly as it should be even when we can't see clearly in the moment, day, month, or year?

Forty-One
Friends

Another large life move meant a new flood of comments from friends and family. This time we were moving in the direction society approved of, so it was less difficult to field the comments. Of course we got the question of whether we were concerned about living together again, but some positive comments from friends who had watched our journey pleasantly surprised us.

"Congratulations to Ryan on getting his PhD!"

"It has been amazing to watch you two support each other's dreams."

"My boyfriend just got transferred to Pennsylvania, and your relationship has given me the confidence that we can get through this."

"I've really seen how you both didn't sacrifice your dreams and a lot of us in our friend group did to some extent. I can see how you will be happier because of that."

"I'm proud of you for making it through these years."

"I'm so happy for you that you will be together again."

"You've inspired me to go follow my dreams because I've seen how you don't let go of yours."

"You gave me the confidence to ask to work remotely so I can see my partner more and do less long distance."

"Watching your journey over these five years has been touching. I know I don't know Ryan, but I've seen how much you love each other and am glad you can be together again."

This time I really only had one answer for everyone. "Thank you."

We didn't need anyone's approval. We had learned to live our life, own our life, and act on what was best for us. The comments no longer pulled me in different directions emotionally because I was confident in my decisions and had healed from the initial heartbreak. I had learned how to love and trust myself more. And wasn't that the whole point? It really was the most important thing I learned and continue to work on; it was endearing to know that someone had observed our path and recognized this evolution. Many had changed their viewpoint on long-distance relationships after watching the sequence of events of our lives unfold. It was a moment in my life where I saw so vividly that we are always leading by example. There is no choice. It's a given. Our actions speak louder than our words. We will create ripple effects, and if we are living in integrity, then we will hopefully create positive change. Most of the time, we never get to know what impact we make and if our decisions have influence. We simply have to trust. Sometimes, though, especially when moving or making a big life change, we are fortunate to hear from others on how we created a positive impression on their life.

I wonder what the world would look like if we shared our thoughts on how someone inspired us as freely as we share our judgments?

Forty-Two

Breaking Free

"Okay, we can finally go to bed!" I let out a sigh of relief. "I have called all my customers and my team twice. Everyone is updated and as happy as possible." I excitedly announced to Ryan. I had prepared my pipeline for the hurricane coming through and I was relieved all procedures were now in place. With the pipeline down for the weather, I was fully convinced this would be my first full night's sleep in weeks.

"Awesome," he replied as he pulled the covers up over his shoulders.

I hopped into bed eager to catch up on some sleep. I was exhausted after the last few weeks of many late-night calls and interviews for other jobs in Virginia. It could've been the location or state of the economy, but I found jobs to interview for that I liked much faster than I had in Los Angeles. It was not lost on me that it was easier because this time I was running toward something rather than running away from it.

I was straddling two worlds with these new opportunities and trying to decide what would be next for me. By this time I had been given several promotions within my company which included a high salary and solid pension and benefits that accumulated by the day. Sometimes the raises made all the calls tolerable . . . but only sometimes. I was trapped by the golden handcuffs and I could feel their grip tightening. I was already looking at a large pay cut to pursue the sustainability work that I was seeking and I could sense that I didn't have much more time before the handcuffs would be too tight to escape.

"Sarah, Sarah." I heard Ryan moan grumpily as he shook my shoulder. "Your phone is going off."

I looked at the time. It was around midnight. I thought for sure we were going to sleep tonight. I had checked all the boxes. How had the peace only lasted for two hours? What had I missed?

It was one of my customers who called frequently. "Hi, Alice," I answered sleepily, grabbing my glasses off the nightstand as if putting them on might make me feel more awake.

"Hi, Sarah!" she nearly shouted, her tone frantic. "Sorry for calling late. I hope I did not wake you!" We both knew this was an obligatory phrase at this hour. I looked at the clock again—it was too late for etiquette.

"No, no it's fine," I mumbled in a deep, groggy tone to purposely clarify that I had been asleep.

"I am calling because the hurricane has started to die down here. It has passed sooner than we expected. I do not know how it is by you, but the winds are pretty calm here. Is it possible to get someone to come out and get flow started to our plant again?"

She didn't know I was in Virginia. The pipeline was very long so she meant the hurricane was calm in Orange County about an hour drive from Houston, but she was not sure how Houston was faring. I let her know that I could not, in good faith, send a technician out in an active hurricane. We needed to wait until the morning to confirm it was safe.

"Okay, are you sure? Because it looks like it has fully passed here," she pushed back on me again.

I sternly reassured her that no one was being sent out in the middle of the night during a major storm.

"Okay, well I had to ask," she relented, with a tinge of irritation in her voice. "I will talk to you in the morning."

I sighed, feeling quite annoyed as I hung up. No one needed to ask about sending technicians out in a storm. These were the kind of calls that should never happen, but they did all the time. They were the product of profit metrics and high performance goals that most employees were under. After some point of losing all normalcy with life and profits on hold in a pandemic, it became an expectation to be able to call around the clock. I could empathize with Alice, doing her best to optimize her production, but I felt angry too. I ended the call and tried to fall back asleep knowing there would be an irksome early morning wake up call waiting for me.

The next morning I continued to field calls between interviews. I was extra tired because Lenny had been ill and we had been to several emergency animal hospitals to find a cure over the past few days. While worrying about him, I had been interviewing for two jobs that could not have been more different. One would exchange the keys to my handcuffs for an equal or even higher salary with expectations to travel often and work some holidays. I even had an interview on Christmas Eve, which spoke volumes of what the expectations might be ahead. The other required a large pay cut to work for a smaller energy efficiency consulting company with an expectation to work standard hours. Originally I was interviewing with them to start a new office in DC, but that office was never constructed. They had decided they still wanted to extend an offer and created a remote role. As I considered my options, my cultural programming made me feel uneasy about taking such a large pay cut. I knew so many people would beg to be in my position. Was I being irrational? Was I throwing away a gift? Was I making a big mistake? My phone buzzed, interrupting my thoughts. I felt the all too familiar tightening of my heart and shoulders at the sound. I looked down to see Alice's number on the caller ID.

My heart quickly spoke up and she reminded me I was searching for happiness and that there was another way; it was okay to go against the status quo. Her voice reminded me that, in the end, I was not looking for either of these jobs. These were both stepping stones to get closer to my dream of opening a yoga studio, which meant work-life balance would be key so I could teach yoga at night. I was, once again, at another life-choice point, a fork in the road with two job offers that would take me in opposite directions. This time I was wiser and more familiar with my heart's voice. I knew from my yoga training that I needed to lead my life by internally referencing and not looking outside of myself for validation on what I should or should not do. I listened. I took a leap of faith and went from a company of seventy-thousand employees to seventy in the pursuit of contributing to sustainability, finding my passion, and directing my life.

I shattered the handcuffs.

And I watched the golden confetti fly.

Forty-Three

Third Heartbreak

Moving back under the same roof as Ryan healed the chasm in my heart, and yet, I quickly found that it also created a new heartbreak I didn't expect. I missed going to Rasa Yoga School. Rasa had been a sanctuary for me over the last five years. It was something in my life that could not be replaced. There are so few places where you can go and know you won't be judged, where the people will greet you with love to welcome you in, at the end of a hard day. I had grown accustomed to seeing my friends and participating in yoga training in person. When I was there, I had yearned to be back with Ryan, and now that I had that, I yearned to be with my yoga sangha (community). It was no doubt a heartbreak. A very different kind, but a heartbreak nonetheless. I truly am so lucky to have had the privilege to have loved so much that it hurt to leave. That is a beautiful gift and I certainly believe that experiencing love and joy is completely worth the heartache it may create.

Right before I left, my mentor Gracie asked if I wanted to have a going away dinner with the teachers. I had always envisioned leaving with a large dinner or party, especially every time I attended events for other students moving away. It made me smile to think about being able to say goodbye to everyone, have some good laughs, and let them know how much they meant to me. Now that I had the chance, I was at another ethical crossroads with COVID. I hadn't gone into a restaurant in six months and I couldn't imagine going at this time. It seemed inappropriate to sit at a table with fifteen people, eating without masks on, when we certainly weren't six feet apart. Saying no to this offer was one of the hardest things I had to decide on; I was deeply saddened. The chance for the going-away celebration was over and I had chosen it. I, of course, will never know if I made the right decision or if there even is a "right" in this case. I had to decide based on the practices I had been following which was to wear a mask and distance to try to slow the spread while hospitals couldn't function. I also didn't want to risk getting COVID right before my flight. It is not always easy to follow principle to the best of our abilities—sometimes life really tests us to see if we are going to stick to our word. This kept my conscience clear, but my heart ached. I felt deflated. I never thought I'd have to turn down a gathering to celebrate my next chapter, and I never thought I'd leave without seeing the majority of my close friends. This left a hole in my heart which has never fully healed.

My sadness was later compounded by the fact that I had trouble meeting yogis and yoginis in Virginia. Normally, my first step after moving would be to go to all the yoga studios and see what is available. This time I had to learn a new way because most studios were only offering virtual options and that didn't lead to meeting people. Plus, I already could take classes virtually with Rasa Yoga, so virtual classes weren't really what I needed. For a short while I did find a studio teaching outdoors, under a tent, within walking distance of our apartment. It was wonderful to be able to leave the apartment and see people! Even if I didn't know them and it was only from a distance. I went to one class where rain was pouring down. The sides of the tent became waterfalls, the top of my mat was soaked, and as we held warrior two I saw the

Third Heartbreak

man next to me get drenched as the wind shifted. We still all enjoyed it immensely because to be outside and sharing a space with people, even in the downpour, was a small moment of bliss. We all needed to get out of the house! Yet this reprieve was short-lived because right before winter the studio announced it would be closing its doors. COVID had led to another local business permanently shutting down. It was sad to see this occur; I know it represented so many businesses and yoga studios that year. I would have to keep finding my way. At least I had met some like-minded people from that studio and one person who even lived at our apartment complex. After I moved, this moment in time felt like I was living in a space of infinite potential, but I didn't know how to tap into it. There were so many people nearby—but how could I connect with them when they were so far away?

Luckily, if the last five years had taught me anything, it was not to fight the situation. I was not going to repeat my old patterns that had played out when Ryan and I were separated. There was no resistance to the distance from the Rasa Yoga community. I let myself feel all the emotions, reassuring myself that they were valid. This time, I would trust that it was in my best interest and that it was an opportunity to grow. I knew moving would help me to master teaching. Now I would need to find my own students and apply the knowledge I had gained. It was the perfect next step in my journey to stand on my own two feet. I could expand into my own as a yogini as long as I could get past the growing pains. And although the chapter had closed where I could step into those doors of Rasa Yoga each evening, I knew it was always just a phone call or plane ride away. As Padma said to me before I left, "This is not a goodbye; you are still part of the community. This is an *until next time.*"

My heartbreak lasted for an entire year. The pivotal turning moment came when I returned to Texas for a yoga retreat with my beloved community. When I arrived, some students had already been there for some time and when I opened the door to the practice room, it was like walking into a wall of pure love. I could literally feel the loving energy of the group in the air as soon as I put my hand on the door. It was surreal to see everyone again and pick up like no time had elapsed. However, for me, time and space had moved on. I was completely overcome by emotion through this entire retreat. All parts of my unhealed wound from leaving were being pried open. I typically sustain a calm demeanor, but I was learning, from the waves of emotion that I was feeling, that I still had a lot of unprocessed emotion from moving away. One day I was overwhelmed by gratitude, and then filled with sadness the next. I would waffle between gratitude and anxiety at any given moment. I had no choice but to give into the vulnerability and allow myself to feel these emotions; they were too strong to hide (especially when I was fasting, meditating, and practicing heart openers on a retreat!!). The ultimate moment of rawness came during a beautiful send off ceremony for a student moving to France. I knew the pain of moving, what she was about to go through, and I was so grateful she had this time with everyone to say goodbye. Since my own grief was still ongoing, this resonated with me and opened my wound big time. There was no hiding from the fact that my heart was wide open and the crying continued. This was a clear indication to me that I had not addressed my heartache enough in the last year. I promised myself I would do two things when I returned home: work on processing these emotions and find a place to teach yoga.

Once home, I did not know how I was going to start to heal and teach, but I knew I was ready; my mind was open to the possibilities. I finally found closure in a private lesson with my teacher Padma, shortly after the retreat. During the lesson, she shared with me that she did not know exactly how to put it, but she had felt more unease in me during the retreat than she was accustomed to feeling from me. I agreed that was the case and I told her about the myriad of emotions I had experienced in those moments. After hearing my explanation, she affirmed my feelings by acknowledging that, looking back, she could see how the way I had to leave so abruptly during the pandemic was extremely difficult and could even be considered a low-level trauma. The word trauma may sound a bit extreme, but it was emotionally scarring to have my life uprooted by a pandemic, live alone for three months, and then fly to another state without saying goodbye to any of the friends or coworkers I had spent every day with for the last five years. Her words of affirmation conveyed that she understood my pain from leaving without a proper goodbye, and they were truly healing. I discovered in that moment that all along I had needed to speak my truth on how I felt in those final days. I had felt unseen and unheard. Shortly after this, I was more at ease and it would not be long before I received many opportunities to teach yoga and meet like-minded yogis and yoginis in Virginia who would become close friends.

Forty-Four

Settled

After making it through our first Virginia winter, we knew we had found our Goldilocks location. Chicago had been much too cold. Los Angeles, mainly because of the lack of AC, but especially Houston, had been much too hot. Virginia, on the other hand, was just right. We were thrilled with the weather, the people, and the beautiful nature surrounding Alexandria, where we lived.

Six months after moving, we decided to find a realtor and buy a house. We went in without a clue that the housing market was ferociously competitive due to COVID. We literally did zero research ahead of time to know that this was a market that highly favored sellers. Our incredible realtor gave us the scoop and I didn't really grasp the gravity of what she was saying. *How bad could it be?* I figured. At our first open house, the seller's realtor was late and as he ran up to the door fumbling for his keys he asked us how long we had been looking.

"Not long. We just started looking recently, and this is our first open house," I said.

"Oh, so you haven't lost on a bunch of offers yet," he replied rather sharply. I stiffened as I sensed an undertone of judgment.

"I do not plan to lose any offers," I retorted in stern, calm, way, my gaze steady. I surprised myself with my answer, but it just came out of me. I was also dead serious. I sincerely did not see us losing an offer.

One month later, we put in an offer on a beautiful house that had been remodeled and was a great fit for us. The best part was, I would finally have a yoga room! In the apartment, I had created a meditation space in the guest room closet, so this was a major upgrade. The kitchen was beautiful and designed well for cooking and hosting. We felt the backyard was serene and a place where we could host bonfires and I identified several spots where I could see Lenny sunbathe. It was far over the budget we had planned on, but we still felt the price was worth it so we went all in. The next day, however, we were informed that we had lost the offer. Someone had bid higher. I couldn't believe it and neither could our realtor. I was confused because I had focused in on this strong inner feeling from the beginning that we wouldn't lose a bid. I thought I had heard my intuition clearly. Still, I was content with letting it go. The market was too inflated, so we decided to wait a year. We didn't need to dive deeper into this insanity.

We had made that choice and had moved on until three days later when our realtor called. "Sarah, I just got a call. The financing on the other offer fell through. The house is yours if you both want it. Are you still interested?"

I was truly shocked. That day we accepted the house. Somehow, in one of the most competitive real estate markets, we had only spent one month and put in one offer to get a gorgeous home in a fantastic neighborhood. This felt incredible after waiting five years to be in the same state.

Six years after graduating college, we were living the life I thought we would live right out of undergrad. We had rewarding jobs that allowed us to be together, a beautiful house, and a cat. We had held onto that dream for over a decade. I thought it was going to be a simple one, but life showed me differently. The length of time it took to get to this point made it all the sweeter, and I was truly proud of us for supporting each other. If we hold onto a vision long enough and make decisions that move us in that direction, the vision will manifest. The road may be winding, we may miss a few exits along the way, but the GPS will keep course correcting for determined minds.

When I look back, the strangest part of being back together in the same place was that time felt like it contracted. It was hard to imagine we were ever apart more than a week or two. I had to remind myself of memories from Houston to grasp that those five years were, in fact, five years. It was like a black hole had created some kind of time warp and what once was an endless stretch of growing pains was just a blip on a screen. The act of being together had healed the open wound. Time really is an illusion. As Emily Dickinson wisely wrote, "Forever is composed of nows." The same event can feel like a lifetime or a blink of an eye depending on our perception. Everything is temporary. We create reality.

Once again I felt the familiar feeling of the cycle: Forget. Remember. Repeat.

After the move, a lot of people asked us if we were finally settled—were we planning to stay here for a long time? I could tell these questions came from a genuine place of curiosity and not from judgment. We had only been in Virginia for a few months, barely knew anything about the area, and had bought a house. I understood why people wondered. Yet all I could say to that question is "No? Not really I guess." I'm not a huge fan of the word settled, and I think that is often *unsettling* for others. To me, it sounds like caving in to comfort over following my heart's desire. Yes, I wanted to live somewhere for more than a year. Ideally, at least five years. But no, I did not see this as our dream home that we had to live our life out in. At the same time, I was open to the reality that it could become a long-term living situation for us. It was our dream and this house was the perfect space when we purchased it. However, completing a dream means that things come full circle and it is time to strive for the next dream. I am certainly willing to move if an unexpected opportunity floats our way. And my ultimate dream is that we never choose to settle. May we always remember to push our boundaries. May we always allow each other to grow. May we always be independent beings who don't need to lean on each other, yet can, when we want to. As Ryan said in his vows, "I promise to make our life an adventure, because adventures always have happy endings."

We reveled in the aftermath of this dream for one glorious year. Lenny was happier than ever, exploring the yard by chewing the grass, talking to the squirrels, meowing at the neighbor's dogs to let them know he was in charge, and chirping at the birds. He asked to go outside constantly and, conveniently for him, the back door was right next to my desk. I'd let him out and watch him bathe in the sun or curl up under his favorite bush while I worked. Then, on one of the worst days of our lives, he was diagnosed with a heart disease where he was given a very short time to live. We started to let him outside more regularly after this diagnosis even though I held onto the hope that he would live a long time and not follow the average statistic of six to twelve months to live. Now it was that much sweeter to watch him be happy, but also heart-wrenching knowing these memories were soon going to be of the past. Over time his breathing became more labored. He did not surpass the somber statistics and we had to face the dreaded day where we said our goodbyes. Lenny transitioned peacefully at our house as he lay in my lap exactly one year to the day after we moved in.

When he came into my life, he gave me a reason to come home for the first time in two years. The house no longer felt lonely, and suddenly, I looked forward to seeing him at the door meowing and giving me a welcome home headbutt. He taught me so much about contentment, love, and trust with how gracefully he lost his old family and embraced his new life with me. The first day I brought him home, he was sick, depressed, and tired. He put his head in the palm of my hand and fell asleep. I promised him that I would keep him safe, I would care for him, and help him heal. I kept to my promise everyday. He returned this by helping me heal each day too. Looking back, I am so grateful that COVID allowed me to have more time with him in what I did not know would be his final years.

On his last day, he once again put his head in the palm of my hand and fell asleep. I could see that he was just as tired as the day we met, but this time he was happy, we had created a deep bond, and my heart hurt because I could not promise to help him heal. We had both rescued each other and now we had come full circle. His love bridged the gap for me while Ryan and I were apart, and I provided him a safe space to recover. Then he came with me from Houston to Virginia to create this new life and complete our dream. He adored having two humans to dote on him and we loved learning how to care for him together. When he passed, it felt like the death of my Houston journey. Endings can be very painful and this one certainly was as these years encompassed so many transitions, moments of growth, sorrows, and joys. At the same time, I was comforted to know that there cannot be an ending without a beginning and that no matter how emotionally difficult an ending may be, the beginning has endless potential.

Lenny was my angel on earth and now he is my angel in heaven.

His passing closed this chapter of my life.

Part Five

Closing Reflections

The longest journey you'll ever take is the eighteen inches from your head to your heart.

—UNKNOWN

Ryan and I had just gotten our driver's licenses after our seventeenth birthdays, which are only four days apart. I felt a new level of freedom and was ready to explore. I held up a map of all the farms in northern New Jersey and asked Ryan if he would visit them with me. Naturally he looked surprised to see that I had picked such an unusual trip, but he, too, is a foodie who loves the outdoors so off we went. It was not actually the right season for vegetable picking, but it was an absolutely picturesque, sunny day in New Jersey to go for a ride. All the addresses for the farms were strategically placed right off the road so that people driving by would see the farm stands full of food, except for the last one. The GPS kept telling us to take turns until it led us down a winding road that eventually went from asphalt to gravel. As we kept being instructed to proceed ahead, we wondered if we should turn around. We had seen enough farms, but quitting was not really in our nature and besides, what if this was the best farm yet? My fear of missing out was strong in high school. Eventually, the GPS announced that we had arrived at our destination and as we peered out the front windshield, all we saw was a residential home. I began to scan the yard for a sign of a farm. My eyes settled on a cobbled stone water well in the middle of the yard. On the front, as clear as day, in dark gray stone were the letters S. DeBlock. I stared for at least ten seconds to make sure my eyes were not tricking me. Then I looked over at Ryan, "Do you have family over in this area that I do not know about?" I asked. He had extended family in New Jersey, so I was thinking it was possible.

"No," he very confidently replied, while he, too, stared at the letters.

We were both speechless. We sat there in stunned silence while staring at the well. After the initial shock wore off, we both agreed it was time to go home. To this day, I still reflect back on this moment with wonder and awe. Where were we and how did the GPS bring us there?

It was all always meant to be.

Forty-Five

Opposites Heal

As I finished writing the first draft of this book, our thirtieth birthdays had just passed. Since we are only four days apart in age, we often refer to our birthdays together, and we have now officially been together for half our lives. My heart is full and overjoyed to reflect on how far we have come, and also because I know our adventure is just beginning.

Writing this book ended up being more therapeutic than I ever anticipated. If there was any lingering discomfort around our decision to live apart, it has vanished through the process of placing words on these pages. I was able to fully forgive myself for not following my heart when making the decision of where to work and accept the way life unfolded. In this way, writing this book was already worth it because it helped me heal, but I started writing this book with the hope that at least one person who may be going through a similar situation can learn from my story and suffer less than I did. This is still my hope.

When I set out to write this piece of my story, I thought this would be an important topic for young couples experiencing distance with dual careers. I thought it was a growing need with more and more people facing this dilemma in a global world. The truth is slightly more nuanced than that, though. Since starting to write, I have learned that many couples in a variety of situations have spent time away from each other, and many more than I realized. It has been a source of pain for couples for decades—just not often openly discussed. I have heard from so many people how distance has been such a relevant topic in their lives that, at some point, it caused unease in their relationships.

I first realized this is not just a millennial issue one day when I was sitting at a table of ladies aged forty to sixty years old. I mentioned that I was writing this book and immediately, one chimed in, "My husband and I actually did two years long distance. We met in school and he graduated medical school two years before me. We drove between our cities to see each other."

The next person immediately followed, "Yeah, I commuted every weekend for a year and spent my weekdays away from my family to finish my nursing school degree. There was nowhere near our house where I could go to school."

This encouraged another to share, "I used to take care of my girls for six months at a time on a regular basis. My husband was in the navy for twenty years and would be at sea."

"Oh, wow, six months is a lot. I used to take care of our family for three months at a time. My husband worked on an oil rig and his schedule was three months on and one month off," added another. The stories kept rolling. It was so touching to see how, just at this table, so many of us shared this background of managing long-distance relationships. I could feel the heart connection that was being created simply by sharing these stories. We recognize ourselves in others and see the connection. The Bhakti House Band eloquently captures this sentiment in their song "Stories":

Like Jesus, Sidharttha, Arjuna, Sita, Rama

Heroes all have struggles but we can learn from the drama

Those who walked before us

Their stories must be told

They're not just myths and legends from the days of old

The challenges they faced were not just their own

They fought and overcame to let you know you're not alone

Working on this book showed me how many people have been in similar situations and that the lessons I learned are not even specific to long-distance relationships. They are universal truths for any relationship. Especially the relationship I have with myself. In order to have a healthy connection with another person, we have to let go of resistance, be willing to ride the highs and lows, continue to grow, trust the other person, take care of ourselves, let our partners be themselves, encourage each other to go places they may fail, and make sacrifices. When looking back at certain circumstances, it may no longer appear that there was a sacrifice and perceived failures may actually become successes. We have to live in the moment while simultaneously keeping our eyes gazing out over the horizon to make decisions that will lead to lasting happiness. It is through practicing yoga and having a teacher that I was able to open to this larger perspective; to realize that we do not see reality but we see the world through our perspective. Therefore the more expansive our perspective, the closer we come to seeing the Truth. Investing in myself during this time, through having a teacher, allowed me to gain tools for self-realization—and that was the best thing I could have done. I vow to always invest in myself and I hope you will, too, because we all deserve that. I have seen the payoff—fulfillment.

I view relationships like two trees growing beside each other. When healthy, they continue to grow taller while always sharing and observing their journey. Their roots grow deeper with some gentle crossing to make their foundation ever stronger, together. The space they give each other still allows them to sway in the wind and the light to shine down through their branches to the forest floor. This provides nutrients for other life to flourish around them. Squirrels and birds may take comfort in their shelter or play among the branches in delight. The time will always come when they need to lose all their leaves and begin again. They understand the cycle of death gives rise to a new season as they watch each leaf fall to the ground. There is trust that it is a moment of transformation and only a temporary ebb in the flow. In due time, as buds form on their branches, bloom into flowers, and fall to create room for the leaves, the abundance of their shade, fruits, and space will be expansive. Through the storms, they may temporarily lean on each other, but if they lean on each other too much, they may weaken both structures. It can limit their ability to twist in a windy storm or even cause rot to form where they overlap, with time.

Pure love is growing side by side while cheering on the other to new heights. Codependency is leaning on each other too long, allowing the boundaries to get muddled, causing rot and decay. Our journey illuminated areas where I had codependency. Really this is just another way to cope with stress in a less than optimal way. It comes from a place of innocence and can be damaging if not addressed. It is another way to dull our senses, just like overeating or drinking when times get difficult. It is a way to run away from our feelings.

I had to look at my feelings to start to straighten my trunk back up. Then I had to feel my feelings so I could allow myself to expand and reach toward the sun. One thing I noticed consistently throughout this process, is that I often felt conflicting emotions. Happy and sad.

Grateful and angry. I learned that I can feel opposite emotions, often at the same time, and this is part of the complexity of being human. Our feelings are multifaceted. More importantly, I learned feelings do not equal truth. If I feel sad, that does not mean something is bad. If I feel scared, that does not necessarily mean I should stop moving forward. If I feel joyful, it does not mean I succeeded. Emotions are energy in motion, and it simply means to feel and acknowledge the energy that is present. Plus, opposites in themselves are healing. Once we become aware of them, it becomes apparent that opposites are all around us.

Hot and cold.

Success and failure.

Inhale and exhale.

Sun and moon.

Divided and united.

Instead of everything feeling like an unsolvable paradox, we can suddenly see that opposites are always there waiting for when we are ready to heal. We can then start to accept that the paradox does not need to be solved: both sides are necessary. Stability comes from learning to navigate this interplay of opposites we experience in life. Balance is the resolution of opposites where we hit the sweet point of tension, and it is important that this not be confused with eliminating the tension.

Ultimately, it is these opposing forces that make us feel alive. When we stop dulling our senses, then we can feel and notice them, and I believe it's when we feel alive that we are happiest. I gained a sincere appreciation for the importance of opposites and the role they played during this chapter of my life. We cannot know happiness without feeling sadness. We cannot feel our limitless nature without first feeling the frustrations of our limitations. We cannot feel our own pure inner joy without being separated.

Yoga philosophy calls the energy of the opposites that create the universe *spanda*. It translates to sacred tremor. Spanda is the movement or vibration that arises from stillness to create consciousness and matter. It is the space in which balance exists, right at the midpoint between positive and negative charges. Spanda keeps life going and allows us to navigate our outer and inner worlds. It is the pulse of the universe and it is the electromagnetic pulse of our hearts. And ultimately, it is this sacred tension that lets us know we are alive. We may mistakenly think we are seeking relief from this tension, but, if we do, we can not feel our full power. When we have the capacity to remain in this sacred tremor, then we can hear and follow our hearts.

Relationships are a microcosm of this macrocosm—opposites coming together but not becoming one another. Sometimes to learn this, we have to take some distance apart while still being together to strike the balance. For after all, love is not possessiveness. When leading with pure love, we let our partners dream. We let our partners soar to new heights. My hope for Ryan and me is that we never stop letting each other grow.

So let your partners soar! Let yourself fly! Feel every ounce of being alive!

Life may take us on some unexpected twists and turns. We must trust that these turns are for our own growth. If we can trust the process, they may just work out—and who are we to judge what's wrong and what's right? Everyone's on their own journey creating their story. We cannot possibly know what is best for each person and that is not our job to figure out. I can't help but wonder, *What would the world look like if we stopped judging and simply watched life beautifully unfold?*

Afterword

As I reflect on the journey detailed in these pages, I feel immense gratitude for the life I now live. Seeing Ryan every day is a joy I do not take for granted. Even if our time together is limited to late evenings, we cherish these moments as a gift of abundance.

Since the conclusion of this book, we have adopted two kittens, Ainsley and Elsie, who have grown and filled our home with playfulness and love. Ryan is currently working at the US Naval Research Laboratory as a chemist, pioneering innovations in battery technology for the next generation. He also enjoys coaching kids in rock climbing on the side.

I took a leap of faith and opened Soma Yoga Healing Center in Alexandria, Virginia, following my heart's calling. This dream, like any other, is challenging, as it pushes me to grow continuously. The lessons I learned during our time apart continue to shape my life every day. I am enthusiastic about this path, the incredible people I meet, and the opportunity to evolve through each and every challenge.

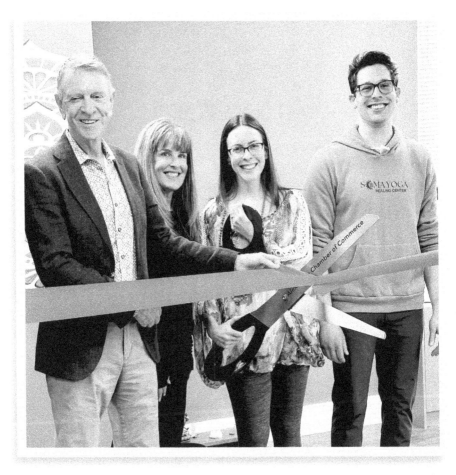

Soma Yoga Healing Center Grand Opening Ribbon Cutting with the Alexandria Chamber of Commerce President, Padma, and Ryan by my side.

Acknowledgments

This book would not have been possible without the support and guidance of many incredible individuals, family members, and friends.

I extend my deepest gratitude to my yoga guru Padma Shakti for planting the seeds of this book. Her encouragement to share my story gave me the courage to embark on this journey and her wisdom continues to inspire me.

I feel blessed to have worked with Jessica Buchanan, a master at memoir writing and a dedicated seeker of self-evolution who generously holds that space for others. Her exceptional skill in bringing out the best in my story, coupled with her developmental editing, has truly shaped this book into what it is today.

I am also immensely grateful to Soul Speak Press for believing in this project and for all of the support to bring it to life.

To my mom and dad, their unwavering love and support have been my foundation. Thank you for always checking in to ensure I had what

I needed, reminding me to believe in myself, and encouraging me to never stop learning.

Thank you to my grandma for joyfully joining me on this journey, reading all the drafts, and providing valuable ideas, such as adding pictures to the book.

And to my husband Ryan, who dedicated countless hours to editing and reading this book throughout its development. His unwavering patience, support, and love are constants in my life that I can always rely on, making all the difference.

Finally, to you, the reader—thank you for taking the time to engage with my story. Your interest and presence give this work its true purpose.

www.ingramcontent.com/pod-product-compliance
Lightning Source LLC
LaVergne TN
LVHW090801230225
804216LV00005B/12